Contents

Introduction

In November 1994, the Maternity Services Group held a two conferences entitled *Listen With Mother: Consulting Users of the Maternity Services*. So successful were they that the Department of Health organized a third conference in July 1995. Edited papers from the conferences are presented in this collection, as a record of three highly enjoyable and informative days, and in the hope that the many people who could not be found a place may still benefit from the advice and experience of the speakers.

The Maternity Services Group (MSG) is an informal alliance of organizations concerned about maternity care, set up by the Maternity Alliance. It includes the Association of Community Health Councils in England and Wales, the Association for Improvements in Maternity Services, the Association of Radical Midwives, the National Childbirth Trust, the National Perinatal Epidemiology Unit, Outreach (an antenatal and postnatal support group in Deptford, south London), the Royal College of Midwives, the Stillbirth and Neonatal Death Society, Support Around Termination for Fetal Abnormality, Toxoplasmosis Trust and WellBeing (the fund-raising body of the Royal College of Obstetricians and Gynaecologists).

The MSG has been meeting regularly since 1989 to discuss changes in the health services which affect women having babies, and to keep member organizations informed about our respective and joint responses to such changes. Over that time, health ministers and health service guidance have constantly exhorted purchasers and providers to consult users about services and, as a result, we have frequently been approached for help in finding out what women want from the maternity services. With the publication of the Parliamentary Health Committee's report in 1992 and the Government's response in setting up the Expert Maternity Group, culminating in 1994 in *Changing Childbirth*, interest became even more intense.

It appeared to members of the MSG that some health service managers were uncertain about how to consult women or had not been doing so effectively. Furthermore, we felt that we needed to clarify the roles of our organizations in consultation and the limitations on our ability to speak definitively about the needs of women all over the country. We also wanted to be sure that the right people were being asked the right questions, and that those who planned to consult women would do more than ask women how satisfied they were, by involving users in the planning and monitoring of services. It was this desire to influence the processes of consultation which led to *Listen with Mother* being a methodological conference rather than an exposition of women's demands.

The conferences took place in London, Leeds and Bristol and were sponsored by the NHS Executive Changing Childbirth Implementation Team. The target audience was people who were involved in planning or monitoring maternity services, not individual practitioners. Four out of five places were reserved for NHS managers or other NHS staff with a user involvement remit and the rest were allocated to members of maternity services liaison committees or community health councils because of their role in service development.

The conferences aimed to give those involved in the development of maternity services a better understanding of:

- Consultation and public participation in decision-making
- The respective contributions of individuals and user organizations at local and national level
- Strengths and weaknesses of various research methodologies
- Ideas for developing effective and sustainable community links, including with marginalised and otherwise hard-to-reach groups
- Ways in which complaints can be used to improve services
- The role of maternity services liaison committees.

The conferences followed the same pattern and included many of the same speakers. They were chaired by Christine Gowdridge, Director of the Maternity Alliance and Karlene Davis, Deputy General Secretary of the Royal College of Midwives. The morning speakers addressed general issues of consultation and participation by users in the maternity services and were followed by a panel of researchers on methodologies, and discussion. Parallel sessions in the afternoon addressed: qualitative and quantitative methods in practice; ways of involving all sections of the community; and consultation as a continuing process. Speakers included professional researchers and NHS staff and members of voluntary organizations with knowledge of specific client groups or of community development. The MSG is most grateful to the speakers who gave their time free.

The success of the conferences led us to believe that the papers presented would be of interest to many who were unable to attend. The papers in this collection are derived from those presented at the three conferences, and we are grateful to all those who gave us the text of their contribution, which certainly made the job of editing easier. We have endeavoured to reflect accurately the spirit and content of each of the presentations. They reflect a range of views and opinions about what is not after all, an exact science. Unfortunately not every contribution from the three conferences has been included either because texts were not available and eventually because of shortage of space.

We hope that the following papers will assist maternity services' planners and providers as they strive to involve users effectively. It is not a simple task but the development of genuinely equitable, women-centred services are worth the effort.

Rosemary Dodds, Policy Research Officer, NCT
Meg Goodman, Health Policy Officer, MA
Suzanne Tyler, Head of Policy, RCM

The History of 'Changing Childbirth'

Kate Jackson

Virginia Bottomley, the then Secretary of State for Health, in her foreword to *Changing Childbirth* stated 'The next step is to open up the discussions locally and nationally on the changes needed in maternity services'. During the three month informal consultation period that followed publication, there was intense debate about the report's recommendations. Consumer groups overwhelmingly welcomed *Changing Childbirth*, as did the Royal College of Midwives. Other professional groups were more cautious and in some instances, anxieties were expressed about the impact of the report's recommendations on the health of women and their babies.

The report also brought to the surface many of the tensions and fears which have long existed between professional groups, most notably GPs, midwives and obstetricians. The report was perceived by some as a charter for midwives - designed to empower the midwife so that she could reclaim her role as an independent autonomous practitioner. Some doctors, particularly GPs, seemed to feel that it was a charter designed to minimise or even eliminate their contribution to the care of the pregnant woman and her family. Some obstetricians felt that they would be excluded from the care of women with uncomplicated pregnancies, with their contribution only being welcome when complications or emergencies arise.

The intention of the report was explicitly stated in the foreword written by Baroness Cumberlege: 'Maternity services should support the mother, her baby and her family during this journey with a view to their short-term safety but also their long-term well-being. They should help the woman to enjoy pregnancy and childbirth as positive, life-enhancing experiences.' In essence this was a charter for women. Without doubt, increasing the choices available to them would involve a review of the way that professionals worked, leading to changes, but this would be part of creating a woman-centred service. The primary motivation for the change was not to ensure that any particular professional group had its status enhanced: it was to ensure choice, continuity and control for women.

Choice
The EMG was convinced that women needed to be able to exercise choice with regard to:

- The professional who would provide the majority of their care
- The place where the birth would take place

In order to make appropriate choices, the EMG recognized that women need good access to unbiased information and to be given the opportunity to discuss the choices available with a professional who could provide unbiased research based advice.

One of the issues that arises frequently when the issue of choice is discussed is whether the woman's right to choose should be paramount, even when this may appear to conflict with concerns regarding the safety of herself or her baby. This issue is discussed within *Changing Childbirth* and the EMG concluded, 'We believe that safety, encompassing as it does the emotional and physical well-being of the mother and baby, must remain the foundation of good maternity care.' The EMG stressed that the key objective for both professionals and women was to ensure the best outcome for the woman and the baby, whilst acknowledging that situations do sometimes arise where: 'Although a good outcome to a pregnancy is desired by the woman, her family, and the professionals who care for her, we found situations where there appeared to be conflict.' The report recommends that the background to such misunderstanding be addressed so that such conflicts could be reduced.

If unbiased information is to form the foundation for informed decision-making, it is important to acknowledge that providing it is not without difficulty. The basis of much of the information currently given to women and their partners is often not research based. This is not always because the evidence has not been sought, but because such evidence does not exist.

Much of the information given to a woman will be based, of necessity, on the experience and opinions of the professionals involved.

Within the context of unbiased information and informed consent, there is also a rather interesting debate to be had about how professionals should react when asked their opinion or experience of a certain option, as well as being asked whether research evidence exists to support it. Home birth is probably the easiest issue to discuss in this context. If a woman with an uncomplicated second pregnancy asks her midwife or GP whether home birth is not thought to be less safe than a hospital birth for a woman, then asks 'what is your view or experience of home birth?', would it be in order for the doctor or midwife to respond: 'Well, I've looked after three women in the past year who were all uncomplicated and everything went really well?'.

Most people would probably feel that this is an acceptable response. On the other hand, what if the professional responded (equally honestly and based and his or her experience). 'Well, as you've asked me, I do have to say that the three women I have looked after this year, all with uncomplicated pregnancies, all ended up being transferred to hospital?'

Some professionals and consumers might feel that this negative and atypical experience would have an overwhelming influence on the woman's decision-making and for this reason should not be expressed. It is important that professionals explore how they deal with questions of this type, and for women to appreciate that a professional's views will be shaped by their experiences.

Apart from the issues regarding unbiased information, the EMG also recognised that information must be provided in a form that is accessible to all women, including those who do not speak English as a first language, and those with sensory disabilities. To encourage developments in this area, Changing Childbirth projects for 1994 included those designed to improve the information available to women.

DEVELOPING ADVOCACY AND TRANSLATION SERVICES FOR NON-ENGLISH SPEAKING WOMEN
This project is running at the Homerton Hospital NHS Trust, East London. Funding has been granted for a computer and word-processing package to produce information leaflets in ten different languages.

DEVELOPING INFORMATION ON MATERNITY SERVICES FOR CLIENTS AND PROFESSIONALS
Lambeth, Southwark and Lewisham Health Commission has been given funding to produce a consumer-friendly booklet on local maternity services in order to facilitate choice for women.

Continuity - Improved care for those women at lower risk

One of the criticisms of *Changing Childbirth* has been that it may result in improved care for those women who are already most likely to have the best outcomes. Such criticism overlooks one of the key tenets of the report which is 'to make care attractive to those women who are least likely to use the service.' Chapter Two of the report addresses in some detail the need to ensure that a woman with a more complicated pregnancy receives care that is best suited to her needs. With this aim in mind Southmead Hospital NHS Trust is currently undertaking a project, funded by Changing Childbirth development monies, designed to ensure that women with complicated pregnancies are able to experience the continuity of care and carer which is the basis of many team midwifery schemes. Similar schemes have also been established in other units; for example, King's Healthcare NHS Trust has established a scheme designed to address the needs of pregnant women with mental health problems and Chelsea and Westminster NHS Trust has set up a team scheme for women who have medical problems during pregnancy.

THE LEAD PROFESSIONAL
This concept has caused difficulties in some parts of the country, primarily, I believe, because it has been viewed from a professional perspective rather than from the woman's perspective as described in *Changing Childbirth*. Some professionals believe that the title implies superiority of the lead professional over all others involved in the woman's care and that it will, therefore, engender professional rivalry and perhaps encourage individuals to work in isolation. The definition within *Changing Childbirth* is, however: 'the professional who would give a substantial part of the care personally and who is responsible for ensuring that the woman has access to care from other professionals as appropriate.'

Once professionals look at the term from the women's viewpoint, it is hard to believe that there can be any reason for conflict. The intention is that the woman should be given the name of the person who will provide a substantial part of her care. The challenge and the issue to which professional energies should be addressed is how to establish, a system whereby a woman can be given that name at the beginning of her pregnancy.

WHO WILL BE THE CHOSEN ONE?
Without doubt, a woman should be given the opportunity as far as is practicable, to choose who will care for her. Unless she knows all the individuals who may be available to care for her, it is likely that she will make her choice on the basis of who she meets first, rather than seeking out a named individual.

What is particularly important is that the woman knows the skills that each professional is able to offer, that she has a realistic picture of her needs and that she is given the appropriate advice and information to allow her to make a decision. A woman's previous experience is likely to influence the type of care she wants. For example, a woman with a previous history of infertility, who has been under the care of a gynaecologist, may wish to be cared for by that person whilst pregnant. A woman with a previous, uncomplicated pregnancy and delivery may wish to be cared for by a midwife, by her GP or both.

On some occasions, a woman may choose to be cared for by a professional who does not feel that they are the appropriate person to provide total care. This is sometimes seen, for example, when a woman who has had a previous lower segment Caesarean section requests a home birth and wishes to be cared for solely by a midwife. In my experience, when this happens, the best outcomes can be achieved where the woman's choice is respected (given that she has had a full and informed discussion with the midwife) and the midwife is supported by the woman's GP, her local supervisor of midwives and an obstetrician. Such support does not require the physical presence of the doctors involved but they should be available and accessible to the midwife should she require advice during the time that she is caring for the woman. The least acceptable outcome is one in which the woman and the midwife are marginalised by other professionals and support and advice are absent.

Control
The need to feel in control of what is happening or what could happen is expressed by many women and such control should be seen as the right of women using the maternity services. However, anecdotal evidence cited by many professionals often points to a large group of women who want professionals to make decisions on their behalf and who are happy to hand them total responsibility for their care. Such anecdotal evidence is not supported by some of the larger studies undertaken in this area. Green's [2] work doesn't support this view and suggests that women wish, at the very least, to be kept informed of what is happening to them, with a substantial proportion wishing to be actively involved in the decision-making process.

Involving users in service planning, development and monitoring

It is apparent from visiting many units throughout England, that consumer involvement is a concept that many purchasers and providers find difficult to incorporate into their organizations. Some, in an attempt to justify the absence of consumers or lay representatives within their planning and development teams, will argue that it isn't possible to find anyone who is truly representative of the local population. This is obviously true, one person cannot represent all interests and this is why purchasers and providers have to look for more imaginative ways of involving local users.

MATERNITY SERVICES LIAISON COMMITTEES

The EMG, recognising the potential difficulties that could occur stated that 'Purchasers should ensure that effective Maternity Services Liaison Committees with proper lay representation including a lay chairperson should be established.' In order to enhance the contribution of the lay members, Changing Childbirth development Monies have been used to support a project run by the Greater London Association of Community Health Councils' designed to provide support, advice and information to lay members of these committees.

Similarly, in order to 'ensure that individuals who do not normally take part in formal consultations are more actively involved', Coventry Health received monies to establish focus groups working with women who are sometimes considered 'hard to reach.' These might include: women from ethnic minority groups, women who are homeless and very young pregnant women.

INVOLVING CONSUMER GROUPS

Consumer groups are often accused of failing to represent all interests, a criticism which they acknowledge and recognise. We must accept though, that it is unrealistic to expect any one group to represent the views of all service users and it is also unfair to reject any suggestions or criticism that the group may make, on the basis of their alleged non-representativeness.

Peter Campbell writing on behalf of the organization Survivors Speakout, states 'if a nursing practice is highlighted as being downgrading or demeaning, does it become less so because my organization has only 50 members? And even less so because they are all over 63 and live in Hendon?'[3].

This quite neatly encapsulates a key issue - when criticised, it is easier and less threatening for the health service to respond by questioning the authority or representativeness of the person (or group) raising the issue, than to look at whether the issue is a problem which needs resolution.

As we look at the developing maternity services, it is easy and perhaps comforting to believe that there is a group of people who know how to get it right, and the main challenge is informing those who are either unaware of the changes that are required or are unwilling to implement them. To an extent, this may be true, but it is probably more helpful to reflect on our own behaviour and identify when and how we have got it wrong, and how as individuals we can improve the situation locally.

On a personal level, I still recall with embarrassment a project which I led, which was designed to improve the uptake of antenatal care for a refugee community living within an area for which I had responsibility for maternity services. The women seemed reluctant to use the hospital antenatal clinic for a variety of reasons including a fear of being reported to the immigration authorities, lack of knowledge, or because they were not registered with a GP.

As a result, they were often seen by a professional for the first time either late in pregnancy or in labour. I thought to improve on this situation by establishing our first 'midwives only clinic' in a community centre used by the refugee women. When a midwife had been allocated to run the clinic, and suitable back-up facilities agreed, I went along to meet the managers of the community centre to explain the plan.

The response was not as I expected. They were neither welcoming nor appreciative of the proposals. They felt that we had made the plans without consultation, we had not spoken to the women involved to find out why they were not coming to the clinic, that we were trying to marginalise those women by offering a second-rate service, and finally, that we were failing to address the central problem: the inflexibility and unwelcoming nature of the hospital antenatal clinic. I had made these plans with the best of intentions but by totally failing to involve the women who would be affected by them, I had caused further problems rather than achieved the desired solutions.

Conclusion

We will only know whether *Changing Childbirth* has achieved its defined goals by asking the women themselves. *Changing Childbirth* does not offer a blueprint for the perfect service which once established will be able to function unchanged for the foreseable future. Successful implementation should mean that in five years' time, we have a service which is sensitive to women's needs and is able to respond with relative ease to the changing demands and expectations of the childbearing woman and her family so that another period of radical change like that through which we are now passing will not be required again.

Kate Jackson
Director Changing Childbirth
Implementation Team

References

1. Department of Health (1994). *Changing Childbirth*. London: HMSO.
2. Green, J. M. et al. (1988). 'Great Expectations: A prospective study of women's expectations and experiences of childbirth', *Child Care & Development Group*, Volume 1. University of Cambridge.
3. Cross, S., Beresford, P. (1993). *Getting Involved, A Practical Manual*. - Open Services Project, Tempo House, 15 Falcon Road, London SW1P 2PJ.

Measuring the Public Voice: Challenges and Pitfalls

Margaret Martin

Introduction

Many years ago when I had been a Community health council Secretary for only a matter of weeks, I was taken on my first visit: to see the maternity unit at the local RAF Hospital. It was a masterpiece of order: babies' cots were at exactly the same place at the end of each mother's bed, everywhere smelt of polish, the mothers were smiling, midwives walked up and down with solicitous but determined steps. I was impressed. And when we spoke to the mothers, they thought it was great as well. The food was wonderful and this was where they had always had their babies.

Coming back in the car, my colleague who was a very active National Childbirth Trust (NCT) member was quiet and serious. 'Well', I said 'there's no doubt about how much the mothers appreciate the care they're getting there'. 'That's because they are not aware of other kinds of care,' she said.

This was my first experience of the complexity of assessing 'the user view'. Since then I have worked with and within consumer organizations, and most recently have been responsible for devising, with purchasers, a strategic framework for involving their local communities in the planning and delivery of services.

I have worked with a team of experienced researchers who are senior social scientists to do this. There are some pertinent lessons to share with you from that work.

- Do *expressed* needs always reflect *real* needs and concerns?
- *Whose voice* do we listen to?
- Do we have clear *aims and outcomes?*
- How do we reconcile different views on *evidence?*
- What are the appropriate *methodologies?*
- What is the impact on the *organization?*

Many managers who will be both commissioning and responding to research on how women want their maternity care provided are generalists: directors of purchasing, customer services, chief officers of public representative organizations. Knowledge of sound research methodologies and social science perspectives is still relatively poor in the NHS. The powerful body of knowledge within specialist organizations stems from detailed, sound research and the single-mindedness of its focus. Yet there are wider issues which they also need to address if they are to change purchasing and provision.

Do expressed needs always reflect real needs and concerns?

Porter and McIntyre[1] have shown in their research on maternity care that user preferences tend to be shaped by what is available. Listening to user views must always be seen as a dialogue with service users in which information in its broadest sense is the key currency. It is a tribute to the stamina of organizations in the field of maternity care that research and user experiences have been the spur to considerable change and to raising women's expectations. *Changing Childbirth*[2] is only the latest in a long line of similar documents and research which highlight how women want their maternity care provided. In an article in the Health Service Journal of February 1994, Lynda Brookes and Mary Black summarise the research on user views over the past few years in a way which clearly illustrates the gap between what women want and what they often get[3].

In addressing this gap we will also need to recognise that people's preferences are shaped by what they know. Their expressed needs will not always reflect their real needs and concerns. The methodologies we use to tap into user views will need to be based on the sound social science perspectives which will enable us to explore this difference.

Whose voice do we listen to?

- Users of a specific service - current/past/future
- Relatives/partners (for their own needs and in relation to their partner)
- Representative organizations - generalist e.g. CHC, specialist e.g. NCT
- Professionals
- Management/policy makers
- General public

Current and past users have a different, more altruistic stake than future users, but it is clearly the case that their perspective changes services for the future. Ensuring that the views and expectations of potential users of maternity services are taken into account has been little explored. The concept of informed views often lies behind our judgements as to whose voice we feel has the most weight in the decision-making process. If current and past users' views are to change the service for future users, then ways must be found for these people to share their experience and expectations.

Locating the individual or user group within the wider society is crucial. We know that racism and sexism in our society are manifestations of the inequality which is deeply rooted in our structures. Because of this we will need to give special attention to the way we seek the views of people from black and ethnic minority groups, as well as those whose disability will challenge the way in which we invite them to participate. There is a host of literature on this and we will need to seek out users' views in different ways. For instance, NW Anglia Commission, in conducting research on the health needs of its Kashmiri community, began by ensuring that the researcher spent at least a month simply living with the community before designing the research[4].

User representation groups will, even in 'alliance', often hold different interests and perspectives: some will have professionals as members, others exclude professionals.

The question is not how representative these groups are (how representative are managers?) but how we address the need to pull together all these different perspectives in a representative way.

What about the wider public interest? On the assumption that everyone's access or improved access to care affects someone else's, there has been considerable interest in involving the public in actively choosing the priorities to which resources are allocated. In reality, though, Oregon-type priority setting exercises have nowhere been found to be very useful. Priority setting is highly complex, and the state of current knowledge of effectiveness suggests that we should view it with caution. We have not even begun to share the effectiveness debate with the public; perhaps because we have not yet shared it amongst ourselves. Choices are rarely simple ones and we need to invest in a better understanding of public values before we can explore public priorities.

The professional perspective can easily dominate this process. Existing teaching and medical education models are only beginning to include psycho-social skills, communication (including cross-cultural) and equal opportunity considerations. Maternity services liaison committees (MSLCs) could provide a real opportunity to encourage a more equal dialogue, but their membership and roles will need to be clarified and strengthened. As they currently exist, most are unequal partnerships and are ripe for review.

Do we have clear aims and outcomes?

It would be rare to find any organizational and individual objectives within the NHS which exclude responsiveness to users. Initiatives like the *Patient's Charter* not only require services to be responsive but actively to promote choice. However, it is often the case that familiarity with the rhetoric deceives us into thinking we are really clear about what we are trying to achieve. A recent national review of methodologies for public participation which we commissioned in our region, showed that there was little evaluation of whether involving the public actually affected the decision-making process[5] There was considerable potential for legitimisation of health service decisions through selective interpretation of the results. The ethical dimensions to this will be discussed later. The first thing we need to ask is whether we want to involve the public or whether we simply want information about their views. The former will mean recognising this as a continuing process, not a one-off dipping into their views as a 'consultation' on service delivery. We need to spend time understanding one another's values. If we only want information on users' views, then we need go no further than the mass of research already available.

Clarity about aims will also involve us asking:

*   What is our agenda (are there any hidden ones)?
*   What is fixed and what can be changed?
*   Can we respond to the outcomes of this process?
*   What is the position of the various stakeholders?
*   What are the appropriate methodologies (taking into account resources, time scale etc.)?
*   How will we know when we have succeeded?

This can be a very searching process. Listening to the public changes people and shifts the balance of power. These processes will test organizations to reflect on their own strengths and weaknesses, to probe current opportunities and identify likely threats and barriers. Another key test for organizations has been highlighted by Allday[6]: the public and users should not only be involved in making decisions about health care and the provision of services, but they should also be involved in:

- Setting the research agenda
- Designing the research
- Conduct of the research
- Analysis, dissemination and implementation

Involving users at the outset in this way inevitably raises expectations. Organizations will need to be committed from the outset to give a clear account of why they are or are not responding to the research findings on user preferences and expectations.

Realism about success is important. We must always question whether any consultation with the public is better than none, and it may be ethically unsound if it raises unrealistic expectations. As Barnes and Wistow[7] have suggested:

'The transformation of relationships between providers and users must not only start somewhere; it must also start at a point where implementation appears to have a reasonable chance of success.'

How do we reconcile different views on evidence?

In an excellent article *Who's afraid of the randomised controlled trial,* Ann Oakley[8] sets out the whole critique of what counts as 'knowledge': the medical model of clinical evidence depends on the randomised controlled trial as the evaluative tool within medicine, the gold standard. Over the last 20 years, however, a new critique has emerged towards what counts as 'knowledge' and there is now a heightened awareness of the importance of designing research strategies which address both the natural and social sciences. However generalist we are, I think this is an area we should be aware of, even in the most basic way.

I listened recently to a Director of Public Health addressing a conference on clinical effectiveness, who referred to 'the danger of consumerism' which could contaminate the effectiveness agenda. Managers are often confronted with the authority of the evidence appearing to conflict with the authority of those who pronounce on matters of public policy. We should be prepared to challenge both. Many of us have seen the effectiveness of alternative therapies or techniques which are not amenable to measurement by randomised controlled trials. There is an added incentive to ensure that social and psycho-social factors are part of the evidence when decisions are made about which care options will be made available. This is particularly true for maternity care, especially if making choices is to be encouraged.

The additional assumption of the medical model, and this is the so-called 'danger of consumerism', is that the user view is diametrically opposed to the medical view. This is not the case. Women are just as interested in safety as the obstetricians are but their experience of childbirth is mediated through a whole host of cultural and social perspectives as well. The debate about the relative safety of the GP-led and midwife-led maternity units, especially the work of Campbell and Macfarlane[9], shows without any doubt that the medical evidence does not support the view that these units are less safe than consultant-led units.

The significance of organizational perspectives such as that of the Association for Improvements in Maternity Services (AIMS) in challenging the view that obstetrics is a scientifically-based speciality, is that this could be applied to the whole of medical science. The work on clinical effectiveness pioneered by the Centre for Health Economics has shown that only 30 per cent (at most) of medical interventions have been evaluated.

However, the empirical high ground is not always restricted to the professions. There is a danger that the 'lay-expert' perspective can adopt the same view about the rightness of its own position. The only realistic way forward is to develop a dialogue which recognises that both perspectives have their own validity or authority. This is an organizational not a methodological challenge.

What are the appropriate methodologies?

Bearing in mind the limitations of the notion of evidence, it still remains true that the weighting (or lack of it) given to broader social and psycho-social factors suffers from poor research methodologies. The emphasis in the past on satisfaction surveys is thankfully waning, and the need to use a wide range of methods, both qualitative and quantitative, is beginning to be recognised in the NHS, largely as a result of the pioneering work of researchers like those who will be addressing you later today. It is also the case that poorly-planned and inappropriate research has been conducted by lay organizations and has been met with cynicism about the value of the user view. No-one can afford to be complacent here.

Research on people is different from research in the natural sciences. Given the dominance of the medical model, it is imperative that we employ experienced social scientists whose professional judgement about the choice and range of methodologies will be sound and their findings will stand up to rigorous scrutiny. From our experience in East Anglia, two points emerge:

- A combination of qualitative and quantitative methods can ensure that the results reflect a deeper understanding of public values and an appreciation of the public's agenda (qualitative)
- They are generalisable to the wider community (quantitative).

Some of the qualitative work we have done has involved focus group work with members of the public. This, in particular, has enabled us to explore feelings and emotions as well as views.

We need a new breed of researcher with all the academic skills but who is also familiar with the wider management agenda and the complex political infrastructure in which managers operate. Dependence on epidemiologists alone in relation to health needs assessment has often resulted in a tendency to focus on quantitative methods, to the detriment of the broader, reflective data which qualitative methods can elicit.

We also need researchers who will challenge us on the ethical grounds of our research. As I said earlier, raising public expectations unrealistically is ethically questionable. So is the more familiar scenario of commissioning research which will not ultimately change a decision; an example would be the closure of a unit since the decision was always going to be made on financial considerations. We experienced this recently with the closure of Newmarket Hospital near Cambridge: despite the continuing claim that the closure was related to issues of safety, financial savings were the ultimate determinant.

There are also ethical considerations in relation to the individuals surveyed. Asking the public to participate in a poorly designed research project is a waste of their time and resources. The costs of participating will be greater than the benefits of the research if the results are questionable and therefore not useful. A competent researcher will have the social skills to treat all individuals involved with respect, to ensure voluntary, informed consent and to ensure that the subjects are appropriate for the study. All our public involvement research in East Anglia has been through research ethics committee approval. The discipline of thinking through the ethical implications of a piece of research is often helped by this process, although researchers do differ as to whether research ethics committee approval is necessary for all social research.

What is the impact on the organization?

Let us imagine that you have thought out your aims and objectives, engaged all the stakeholders, employed the broader-based researcher to work with you: what then?

Why, we ask, is so much excellent research still on the shelf? The Black Report[10], for example, has yet to have much impact beyond academic circles. The political realities can overwhelm research realities. There is also a long-standing failure of health service research to address the factors which inhibit and facilitate change in the NHS. It is often all 'R' and no 'D'. 'Learning by doing' is the key to organizational learning, and we need to emphasise that a strong commitment to development will have to be part of the design of research programmes. The current model is predominantly that of dissemination rather than development. The test of the Cochrane Collaboration[12] and similar exercises will be to see if there is evidence that these reviews are used by clinicians to guide their practice.

When new ways of thinking, new circumstances, new structures begin to flood in, the establishment creaks, sways and groans and settles in precarious positions. The processes that people will need to go through - from questioning, to shared questioning, to confusion, to consensus will take time. We need to give change space to happen, and the organizational supports must be there: the no-blame culture, challenging norms. Relinquishing belief in the rightness of one's practice or standard is hard for anyone because to change those actions, they have to change themselves. Users fear professional retaliation: professionals fear that users will deny professional expertise and power to do good. The process of negotiation needs mutual respect and a recognition that underneath all the discomfort there is a common commitment to the best interests of the public who use and fund our health service.

Margaret Martin,
Formerly Assistant Director
Information and Development
Anglia and Oxford Regional Health Authority

References

1. Porter and McIntyre (1984). 'What is, must be best', *Social Science & Medicine*, 19, pp.1197-1200.
2. Department of Health (1993). *Changing Childbirth*, London: HMSO.
3. Brookes, L., Black, M. (1994). 'Local delivery', *Health Service Journal*, 10 February, p.33.
4. N W Anglia Health Commission (1994). *Health Needs of the Kashmiri Population in Peterborough.*
5. Hamilton Gurney, B. (1994). 'Public Participation in Health Care: Involving the public in health care decision making: a critical review, Health services Research group', University of Cambridge.
6. Allday, L. (1993). 'Shaping the structure of the NHS - a consumer perspective', NHS Executive (unpublished).
7. Barnes, M., Wistow, G. (1992). Researching User Involvement, Nuffield Institute for Health service Studies.
8. Oakley, A. (1990). 'Women's Health Counts' ed. Roberts H.
9. Campbell, R., Macfarlane, A. (1995). 'Where to be born?: the debate and the evidence', Oxford: NPEU.
10. DHSS (1980). 'Inequalities in Health, report of a working party', London: HMSO.
11. The Cochrane Collaboration, P.O. Box 777, Oxford OX3 7LF.

Learning From Experience

Marcia Kelson

Introduction

The aim of all College of Health work is to give people the information they need to make the most effective use of the health service and to improve the quality and quantity of communication between health service professionals and patients.

The *Changing Childbirth* [1] report was welcomed by the College, not least because it places the woman firmly at the centre of decisions about her care. It provides clearly stated objectives and action points for bringing about change. The report also acknowledges the need to involve consumers fully in service planning, in drawing up specifications and quality standards and in monitoring activities. Consumer involvement is advocated not only at an individual level but also at a collective level. For example, *Changing Childbirth* supports consumer groups in playing an active role in assessing services on behalf of women using them, and in working with purchasers and providers to bring about change. The publication of the report represents a significant milestone because it provides a basic framework for future developments.

Efforts to turn the rhetoric of consumer involvement into practice are the focus of this conference and in that context I would like to tell you about some work I have been doing on behalf of the consumer subgroup of the Clinical Outcomes Group (COG).

COG is an advisory group chaired by the Chief Medical Officer and the Chief Nursing Officer that aims to promote effective and efficient clinical practice. The remit of the COG consumer subgroup, members of which are drawn from organizations with a significant patient interest input, is to clarify the existing involvement of consumers in clinical audit and to develop that involvement in consultation with COG.

Earlier this year, I produced a report [2] on behalf of the subgroup which reviewed developments and issues of good practice in consumer involvement across the whole spectrum of the health services. Some of the issues that emerged are of direct relevance to maternity services. This paper discusses some of these.

Modern clinical practice recognises that patients are not merely passive recipients of advice and procedures from health professionals. Rather, they have an active role to play in their care and have opinions about the ways in which health services are provided and may be improved.

In recent years a number of developments have reinforced the position of the consumer on the NHS policy agenda. Policy documents, including the 1989 White Paper [3] the *Patient's Charter* [4] and *Local Voices* [5] have contributed, emphasising the consumer's right to information, to a quality service and to a say in the ways in which services are provided and delivered. The *Changing Childbirth* report could be added to the list.

In 1995, therefore the consumer is firmly placed, in principle at least, on the health service policy agenda. There is also evidence from specific developments: the Patients Forum meets regularly with the NHS Patient Empowerment Focus Group, the NHSE has its own Quality and Consumer group, and increasingly includes representatives from patients' organizations in its working parties and advisory groups; the royal colleges increasingly involve users (both individuals and user groups) as members of patient liaison groups and in specific initiatives. The Royal College of Obstetricians and Gynaecologists Consumer Forum, for example, includes consumer organizations, especially those with a particular interest in maternity services. To date, the Royal College of Midwives has no formal patient liaison group, although it works closely with voluntary organizations in many ways.

Aside from national initiatives, providers and purchasers have posts with specific responsibility for creating and developing consumer involvement initiatives locally. Many of those involved in the maternity services, both purchasers and providers, are making efforts to implement the *Changing Childbirth* proposals on user involvement.

However, despite all these apparently laudable activities, I believe that the published literature on user involvement across the whole gamut of health service provision, raises a number of fundamental questions which relate to how to put the theory of user involvement into practice. Three specific issues emerge: the why, who and how of user involvement.

Why user involvement?

Even assuming that health service professionals are committed to user involvement (and by no means everyone is convinced), the objectives differ both between individuals and organizations within them. Researchers at Portsmouth University[6], for example, recently identified a range of different objectives for different health commissions, including:

- Informing the public about health issues and concerns
- Establishing accountability to and credibility with local communities
- Seeking feedback on current services and future needs

The authors argued that, in the absence of clear and comprehensive organizational strategies, public involvement is a 'pick and mix' approach.

Other authors have made similar observations about user involvement at the provider level. Specific criticisms of user involvement in clinical audit relate to the fact that initiatives tend to be one-off exercises rather than an ongoing feature of audit activity.

Who to involve?

There remains a considerable problem in deciding *who* to involve. *Whose* voice do we listen to?

Who you consult with will depend to some extent on the aims of the initiative. Even in maternity services, there is a wide range of potential consumes to engage: current users, partners, potential users and user representatives who may be user generalists, for example CHC members, or specialists such as the National Childbirth Trust. If specialists are consulted, are attempts made to canvass the views of groups not necessarily represented by that specialist group? What about non-English speakers, mothers with learning difficulties or teenage mothers, for example? Are concerted attempts being made to involve them as regularly and systematically as their more vocal and perhaps articulate counterparts? It may be necessary to draw on a wide range of individuals and/or groups to avoid unrepresentative or tokenistic user involvement.

How to involve users?

The consumer involvement literature covers a confusing array of methods, ranging from patient satisfaction surveys, through public consultation meetings and consensus conferences to more qualitative methods using open-ended interviews, discussion and focus groups.

The choice of methods may often appear somewhat arbitrary: it is rarely clear why certain methods have been chosen or rejected in favour of others. A large body of literature has been built up criticising initiatives which employ inappropriate methods. including the commonly used patient satisfaction questionnaire.

At issue here is not the use of patient satisfaction studies *per se* but the fact that they do have to be well designed and properly administered to produce results that will positively influence the process and/or product of patient care. Staff who are expected to set up surveys are not necessarily adequately trained in questionnaire design, sampling and data analysis. Asking users how satisfied they are usually produces a high overall satisfaction rating. This fails, however, to reflect concerns expressed by patients when permitted to elaborate on individual topics. If you are really interested in finding out what needs changing, it may be more fruitful to ask patients 'what happened to you?'. Leading questions such as 'what went wrong' or 'what were the worst aspects of the service, your care etc.' will probably provide even more revealing insights into the real experiences of users.

Patient satisfaction surveys are also frequently criticised for the top down approach usually employed in their design, administration and analysis. They are more often than not designed by health service professionals to answer questions posed by health professionals, and the results are used to implement the changes that the health service professionals consider most important. This is not a good model for active user participation, but it continues to be the method most widely used to canvass patients' opinions.

Levels of involvement

The majority of reported initiatives fall into the passive end of the scale, while the rhetoric, including that of *Changing Childbirth*, demands more active input.

At the College of Health, colleagues have developed consumer audit[7] - a methodology using a range of qualitative techniques for obtaining feedback from patients about healthcare services. The emphasis is on looking at services from the patient's point of view. In-depth semi-structured interviews and focus groups help identify what patients, partners or carers and potential users think of services and want from them.

Users can be involved at different stages of clinical audit:

- At the start of the study, meetings are held with users, carers and members of voluntary and patient organizations to find out what they think the issues are, and this informs the design of any interview schedule.

- Audit steering groups can include members of user and carer groups, the CHC and so on, as well as purchaser and provider staff.

- User group and CHC members can be trained to conduct interviews with patients and feed results back.

- Feedback from non-users can provide important information about access to services, referral practices or perceived quality for example. In the care of maternity for example, it may be revealing to find out why those women who opt for private maternity care do so in preference to choosing the service offered by the NHS.

- User views can be sought not only on content, but also on the formats or media that are most user friendly.

The establishment of MSLCs goes some way towards actively engaging the consumer perspective. However, there is a danger of having achieved a certain degree of success, they then rest on their laurels, waiting for the rest of the health service to catch up. A personal anecdote may illustrate this:

Earlier this week, and knowing that I was coming here, I asked a friend of mine, an NCT antenatal teacher, about her experiences serving on two local MSLCs.

'Did they have lay chairs?', I asked. 'Well, yes', but she sounded a little doubtful. 'Well one of them is an ex-midwife. The other is an NCT antenatal teacher but the medical members seemed most pleased to have her because her husband is a consultant obstetrician in another part of London!'

I asked her about representatives: 'NCT members from each of the branches whose members fall into the catchment area. Non NCT members have no direct representation,' she replied.

I also asked her if there had been any attempts to canvass opinions of minority groups, to provide information or translate surveys into minority languages. The answer was 'no' on each count for both committees.

Had she had any written information detailing the remit or function of the committee, or her own expected contribution to it? Had she been offered any training? 'No' to all, came the answer, although she knew that one of the lay chairs had gone on the Greater London Association of Community Health Councils' course on her own initiative and at her own expense.

What attempts had been made to ask users about their experiences of services? 'Input from the NCT reps and a couple of patient satisfaction surveys,' and 'no', users had not been involved in designing the surveys.

These experiences are likely to be replicated in many other areas and my friend's answers suggest there remains much to be done actively to engage the views of the widest possible community of maternity service users.

The published literature on user involvement includes not only discussion of specific methods but also a number of articles and booklets that provide working guidelines for active and effective consumer involvement. These tend to have been produced independently by providers, purchasers and consumers themselves but essentially similar themes emerge. In particular, they stress the need for an in-built organizational structure and culture with an understanding of and commitment to consumer involvement.

Organizational factors

The guidelines suggest that true consumer involvement can only work when organizations address the key issues of access and support in practical ways: not just in the physical environment - with ramps and so on - but through the provision of information and materials, transport and appropriate timing of meetings. The involvement of some individuals or groups of consumers may be influenced by language, culture or lifestyle differences which the organization must address. The agency also needs to appoint people responsible for developing user involvement who have sufficient status to introduce service users to all levels of the decision-making process. User groups need budgets for meeting expenses, training and administrative costs and it may even be appropriate for user groups to receive fees for consultation.

Summary

Lessons that can be learned from the recent consumer involvement literature include the following:

- Be clear about the aims of any involvement initiative.

- Distinguish between informing users about services, consulting with them or actively involving them as equal partners.

- Be clear about WHOSE voice to listen to, and attempt to engage the so-called 'silent voices'.

- Be clear about the pros and cons of different ways of involving users.

- Use methods appropriate to the aims of the task and for the target user groups.

- Do not assume that user involvement will be readily taken on board. All those involved may need training in the principles and methods of effective user involvement.

This paper has largely been concerned with collective user involvement rather than with individual involvement in decision making. However, I would like to raise a final question relevant to the matter of the ready assimilation of user involvement. At a recent meeting of the Patient Empowerment Focus Group the important point was made that it is all very well talking about providing patients with information and encouraging them to make informed choices, but what happens when the professional and the patient strongly disagree over what action to take? If we are aiming for true partnerships, rather than what has been termed the 'doctor knows best' scenario, how do we determine where the balance of power lies when the key participants are firmly entrenched on opposite sides of the fence? Where treatment options exist, but there is no scientific evidence for the efficacy of one procedure over the other, do we go with the clinician's preferred course of action - based perhaps on his or her training, or simply on selective preference, or do we follow patient preferences?

Such grey areas add to the already complex problems of how to involve users appropriately and effectively in health service provisions, delivery, monitoring, evaluation and change, and illustrate some of the real shifts in thinking, culture and practice that still need to come about if we are to provide appropriate, accessible, efficient and effective care and service.

Marcia Kelson
College of Health

References
1. Department of Health (1993). *Changing Childbirth*. Report of the Expert Maternity Group, London: HMSO.
2. Kelson, M. (1995). 'Consumer Involvement Initiatives in Clinical Audit and Outcomes. A review of developments and issues in the identification of good practice'. College of Health, February.
3. Department of Health (1989). *Working for Patients*. London: HMSO.
4. Department of Health (1991). *NHS The Patient's Charter*. London: HMSO.
5. NHS Management Executive (1992). 'Local voices and the views of people in purchasing for health'
6. Wessex Regional Health Authority (1993). 'Consumer and public involvement in health commissioning: Learning from experience in Southampton and Portsmouth - Southampton Health Authority.
7. College of Health (1994). 'Consumer Audit Guidelines'. London: College of Health.

Consulting Users of the Maternity Services - The Voluntary Organizations

Mary Newburn

'It is unrealistic to expect the impetus for change to come from those who will not benefit from it.... The onus for reform has to come from the users of the service'
Marjorie Tew, 1990. *Safer Childbirth.*

Levels of consultation

Consultation with users of the maternity services happens at three different levels and each of these offers particular advantages and limitations. Consultation can be directly with current users, with local user representatives, or with the maternity organizations nationally.

Local	direct	Current users Personal views and experiences
	indirect	User representatives on MSCLS CHCs, MUGs Personal contacts Local insight Public knowledge
National	indirect	Maternity organizations Professional insight National overview Public knowledge

Table 1: Consultation with users

Current users

The advantage of consulting locally with current users is that they know about and have direct experience of the services; they make up the local community, they can tell you their own needs, preferences and the constraints they face. If they are asked, they are in a position to say what was particularly good or particularly bad about the services provided. Any troubles they have had are real, immediate and often painful. If they trust you enough to tell you, or have enough faith in you to go to the trouble of explaining, you can learn a lot from them.

Current users can talk about local health care at first hand - the choices offered or withheld, the time they were given or denied, the support they felt or the isolation. It is very important that there should be direct feedback on services and that the messages are used in planning future provision.

The most usual way to sound out the experiences and views of current users is to conduct a self-complete postal survey. Those who wish to conduct a survey should use or adapt the OPCS questionnaire designed to investigate women's experiences of the maternity services[1]. It may be useful to compare clinical or social outcomes for different groups of women[2,3], though researchers advise caution in explaining any differences unless a randomised controlled trial has been used, offering one group a new treatment or form of care. This design was used by Flint when she set up the Know Your Midwife scheme at St George's, Tooting[4,] and is currently being used by McGinley at Rottenrow, Glasgow.

Focus groups and patient panels are being used more frequently. They are able to show what people like and dislike about services and why people feel the way they do. Research, which tends to be costly and time-consuming to design, implement, analyse and report on, is nevertheless important. It allows local women to voice their views.

Examples of Projecting Consulting Current Users
One to One Midwifery Care Centre for Midwifery Practice, Queen Charlotte's, London
Midwifery Development Unit, Rotten Row, Glasgow
Maternity Services, Oldham and Tameside NCT, for West Pennine Health Purchasing Consortium
Choices Project, North Essex, NCT

Table 2

Whilst detailed research can only be done periodically because of the costs involved, data collection should become routine. For instance, women who have some particular medical intervention could be asked how they felt about it, and this aspect of care could be considered alongside other aspects of clinical audit. Anonymous, one-sheet feedback forms could be used regularly for, say, antenatal classes or postnatal care in hospital.

Limitations to direct consultation

The costs of direct consultation with service users are considerable and there is a time-lag between designing a study and getting the results. Current users' views will inevitably also be limited by their expectation. For example, when finding out how important it is for women to have care from the same midwife throughout pregnancy, the birth and afterwards, it is important to be aware that the replies women give will be affected by what they believe to be possible, by what they have experienced, and by the quality of care they have come to expect. The lower women's expectations are, the more easily they are satisfied. Current users may also be reluctant to seem ungrateful if they know the staff were overstretched. Women who have had the worst experiences worry that their case could be identified and they fear reprisals, perhaps when next in labour. Furthermore, some users are easier to reach than others. Finding out the needs of particular minority groups may involve working with advocates, translating materials and setting up meetings in a familiar setting.

Local user representatives

Local user representatives have the advantage of being in touch with the area and the people who use the services and yet may have other relevant information about research, about services offered in other areas, or about agreed good practice, such as ways of enabling more women to breastfeed. Because they combine these qualities, they are a very important group to consult. They can be consulted regularly and from their experience and network of contacts they can respond on a range of topics fairly quickly. User representatives should play a central role on MSLCs, contributing to information for users, contract specifications and standards, clinical protocols, audit, and the handling of complaints. They can also contribute to the design and planning of research to obtain local users' views.

The limitations on consultation with local user representatives are that they are overworked and usually unpaid. In many areas women even experience difficulties in getting their necessary out-of-pocket expenses for meetings covered, such as child care and travel. It is not reasonable to expect mothers of young children to come to meetings without reimbursing them for using a childminder or baby-sitter. Although some health authorities drag their feet over this, in one or two more progressive areas, those who give their time to serving on the MSLC are now being paid an honorarium for doing so.

User representatives are more likely to be effective if they have had some relevant training. Many of the NCT representatives have trained, and practice, as antenatal teachers or breastfeeding counsellors, so they know some areas of maternity care fairly thoroughly. The NCT is currently developing training specifically for representatives on health committees, including critical appraisal skills. GLACHC has Changing Childbirth funding to provide support for lay representatives on MSLCs in the London area.

One MSLC in Surrey has a Consumer sub-group with the aim of increasing the contribution from women and their partners who are using the services[5.] Issues raised by the sub-group, such as how the clinic works, an information checklist or the confusion around vitamin K, are fed back to the MSLC. (More details of how this group works are to be found in the paper by Gillian Fletcher.)

The Effective Care sub-group at Camden and Islington Health Authority was set up to concentrate on research-based care. It looks at the policies of the three provider units and encourages audit. Topics prioritised initially are:

1) Corticosteroids for pre-term labour
2) Prophylactic antibiotic for Caesarean sections
3) Material used for suturing the perineum
4) External cephalic version for breech babies

There are three user representatives on the group, which is chaired by one of the purchasing team and reports to the MSLC.

National maternity organizations

Consulting with national maternity organizations also has its place. Though operating on tight budgets, workers at national level are generally better resourced than local user representatives, having access to a specialist library and a range of research and policy literature. National workers may have a broader base of knowledge. At national level, the organizations also conduct maternity care surveys and develop policy themselves. For example, NCT has published surveys on women's experiences of epidurals, rupture of the membranes in labour, postnatal infections and perineal trauma, and in 1991 and 1992 conducted surveys on women's experiences of the maternity services. As another example, SANDS has produced practical Guidelines for Health Professionals[6]. They challenge the assumption that it is only good news parents want to hear. For many parents, they say, it is better to know the truth than not to know.

Can we speak for parents? Sometimes the national organizations are asked whether they can speak for parents. While it is not sufficient to consult only with the well known organizations, we do attempt to represent the parents who never become members. We are aware of the kinds of issues that lead to difficulties for parents, such as poverty, lack of adequate parental leave, poor information, fear of health professionals, centralisation of services, the internal market. Many examples spring to mind, one maternity unit we know of will not distribute the health authority's Choices leaflet to women. The local NHS trust are in direct competition and the unit in question is offering a more limited range of services than its direct competitor. The local women lose out, but how many of them realise there is a leaflet they have not been given?

Examples of consultation with national maternity organizations:
• Priorities for research in the NHS
• Health Select Committee: enquiry into the maternity services
• Audit Commission: survey of the maternity services
• National Perinatal Epidemiology Unit
• Royal College of Midwives
• Royal College of Obstetricians and Gynaecologists
• Health Education Authority
• Department of Health
• *But Will It Work Doctor?*: A conference on involving users of health services in outcomes research, organised by: Consumer Health Information Consortium, the King's Fund Centre, the UK Cochrane Centre and Oxford RHA

Table 3

The kind of in-depth information national organizations gather explains why things happen the way they do, and why women and their partners feel good about their care or let down. If a problem exists for some women it is a real problem. Sometimes, organizations are discounted as being unrepresentative. Make no mistake, if more privileged, more articulate women - the sort who get involved with self-help support groups or are willing to spend their own time on lobbying - get conflicting advice, feel isolated and unimportant, it is highly unlikely that other women don't feel the same way too. They may, however, be too hard pressed, feel too powerless or simply resigned to it, so they don't speak out.

If you have good contacts with a wide range of user representatives locally, you may not need to approach the maternity organizations nationally. Local workers can be your link with the organizations, combining local knowledge with expertise.

The Maternity Alliance, which does not have local members because it is an umbrella organization, works rather differently than the NCT, AIMS or SANDS. It draws on the experience of member organizations and the enquiries it receives from the general public to develop policy and produce publications, such as the 'Birth Plan', 'New Lives' pack, the report on 'Sugar in Baby Foods', or the survey of the experiences of women with a disability, 'Mothers' Pride'.

The best way to find out about new publications and policies developed at national level, if you do not have a local contact, is to subscribe to the maternity organizations' journals. In some cases this means becoming a member. Through reading the journals you will also hear about the topics of current concern to parents and to workers.

The limitations of consulting with the organizations at their national addresses is that they probably do not know your local area, its population profile and history of maternity provision. Voluntary organizations are also seriously under-resourced. To give you some idea of the scale of operations, the NCT has about 25 paid staff at the national office. Most of these are working to support several thousand voluntary and nominally paid workers, in a network of some 380 branches, and total membership of 50,000. Maternity Alliance has eight staff. All the work done by AIMS, both locally and nationally, is done by volunteers.

Resources

The maternity organizations want to contribute to developments in policy and practice and remain solvent. Increasingly, they are developing consultancy arrangements whereby they contribute to policy reviews or provide training for a fee. It is costly to establish and maintain an adequate level of current awareness and expertise. It is crucial to the financial security of the maternity organizations that they pass on the costs incurred in undertaking detailed work, particularly as there is little or no support from central government for core funding these days.

As a rule of thumb, we respond freely to simple requests by raising some key issues. We may suggest some useful reading or relevant models of good practice, but more detailed work is done by arrangement. If you are writing to us, it is helpful to be told whether you already have local contacts and what comments or suggestions have been received from them.

Private troubles, public issues

Consultation is needed to find out about local communities and the constraints on particular groups of women within those communities.

The sociologist C. Wright Mills talked about private troubles and public issues:

> *'A trouble is a private matter: values cherished by an individual are felt by him to be threatened....... An issue is a public matter: some value cherished by the public is felt to be threatened'*[7]

Current users know about their own private troubles, national maternity organizations make it their business to translate these into public issues. Local user representatives, so long as they are from a variety of relevant backgrounds, supported nationally and part of a local community network, should be in touch with local women's troubles and conscious of the broader issues. Most of those working on policy issues at national level in the membership organizations have worked locally on maternity issues first. Their interest and commitment grew from their own experience.

The 'Challenge of Change' is a recent NCT publication, designed to help local groups of women and user representatives on health committees, draw attention to the issues that are important locally and to achieve change. Anyone who wants to find out more about what women are doing and what the NCT is doing to support them, please buy a copy.

Mary Newburn
Head of Policy and Research
National Childbirth Trust

References

1. Mason, V. (1989). *Women's Experience of Maternity Care - A Survey Manual.* London: HMSO.
2. Green, J.M., Coupland, V.A., Kitzinger, J.B. 'Expectations, experiences and psychological outcomes of childbirth: a prospective study of 825 women'. *Birth* 17 (1): pp.15-24.
3. Oakley, A. (1990). 'Social support and pregnancy outcome'. *British Journal of Obstetrics and Gynaecology*, 97(2): pp.155-62.
4. Flint, C. Know Your Midwife.
5. Fletcher, C. Improving Maternity Services.
6. Stillbirth and Neonatal Death Society (1991). *Miscarriage, Stillbirth and Neonatal Death: Guidelines for Professionals.*
7. Wright Mills, C. (1959). *The Sociological Imagination.*

Qualitative Research Methods 1

Christine Roberts

Introduction

Qualitative research is concerned with understanding people and behaviour rather than with measuring them. It asks the questions what? why? and how? but cannot answer the question how many?

Qualitative research methods allow participants to set their own agenda instead of making them respond to one predetermined by a researcher. This is particularly useful when the subject under discussion is relatively unexplored and the possible responses diverse or unknown beforehand or where a researcher wants to explore motivations, attitudes and behaviour. They are best used to:

- Identify a range of behaviour
- Solve particular problems
- Generate hypotheses
- Provide input to a future stage of research or development.

Quantitative methods usually require a highly structured questionnaire and are susceptible to statistical measurement. They are less dependent than qualitative methods on the individual researcher's interpretation of responses. Quantitative methods tend to appeal to the 'decision-makers' in organizations.

Qualitative methods, on the other hand, are flexible and generally use an open-ended interview format. They allow for understanding of process and motivation which means that the individual researcher's interpretation is critical.

Qualitative research projects

Examples of typical qualitative research projects include:

- Awareness and usage of services
- Needs assessment
- Priorities in health care provision
- Attitudes and behaviour regarding health-related issues such as diet and exercise, contraception, breast feeding and antenatal screening
- Development and evaluation of communication material.

Qualitative research methods

There are two main categories of qualitative methods: group discussions and in-depth interviews. Group discussions usually involve about six to eight people drawn from similar backgrounds and recruited to a pre-determined criteria.

For example, this might be first time mothers or pregnant women. The objective is that participants exchange experiences, attitudes and beliefs about a particular issue. In-depth interviews by contrast are done on a one-to-one basis, to explore an individual's behaviour and attitudes. Interviews might be conducted amongst a highly diverse population and are useful for probing intimate or sensitive subjects, or where there is a strong social pressure to conform.

Group discussions and in-depth interviews should always be convened and conducted by a trained and experienced moderator. They usually take about an hour and a half.

The role of the researcher

The researcher's job is to initiate topics and listen both to what is being said and how it is said. She may respond and follow-up by asking non-directive questions and will ensure that all the relevant topics are covered. The researcher also has a role to play in controlling the dynamics of the group and ensuring that there is equal participation by members.

A typical qualitative research project

A maternity unit might wish to test its draft information booklet for women about health during pregnancy, to explore the clarity, relevance and presentation of the booklet and make recommendations for improvements. Qualitative research methods would be appropriate for several reasons:

- To assess lengthy written material
- To allow flexibility of responses
- To explore respondents' feelings and emotions
- To encourage creative thinking and problem solving.

Women would be the core target audience for the booklet so a possible methodology might include eight interviews and eight group discussions with first time pregnant women and new mothers, structured by age, socio-economic status, stage of pregnancy and location. The secondary target audiences of partners and midwives/health visitors might involve eight in-depth interviews with each group.

The possible outcomes of the research might include:

- Identification of difficult words or phrases
- Assessment of the clarity and effectiveness of illustrations
- Identification of sources of information
- Distinction between the concerns of the different target audiences
- Suggestions for a new section or a different focus
- Realisation that the sampling procedures were partial or biased in some way.

Possible pitfalls of qualitative research

Qualitative methods have their drawbacks. Problems arise when groups are dominated by particular individuals, including a moderator unskilled at managing or understanding group dynamics. The moderator or interviewer may ignore important non-verbal communication or may accept comments at their face value, presenting narrative rather than interpretative and analytical reporting.

Conclusions

The nature of the information required should be an essential determinant of the appropriate methodology. Quantitative approaches are not always useful and qualitative data can be just as valid as quantitative data.

Christine Roberts
Researcher with Cragg, Ross & Dawson

Qualitative Research Methods 2

Wendy Sykes

Qualitative research is different from quantitative research in that it takes a flexible approach to individual sample members. In essence, the process of collecting information is conditioned by what people have to say, the issues that are of concern to them, and the individual experiences they have had.

There are two key methodologies involved in undertaking qualitative research. Although different names might be used these are:

- Interviews with individuals
- Interviews with groups of individuals

In an individual interview, the researcher usually has an outline of the broad areas to be covered. This sets the agenda, but is not rigidly adhered to nor necessarily followed in any set order. As the research proceeds, the guide will generally develop and change to cover new issues as they emerge.

Individual interviews allow a detailed and coherent picture of each person's views and experiences to emerge in a setting where sensitive issues can be addressed. This is particularly important when research is covering subjects that are very painful to respondents, or issues where there may be lack of confidence about expressing true feelings in the face of strong pressures to conform.

Group interviews usually involve up to ten respondents. The researcher's main role is to stimulate discussion - once again within a roughly pre-specified framework - and to ensure that the range of views represented within the group is expressed as fully as possible.

The advantage of a group interview is that the group dynamic will often provide a catalyst to disclosure, encouraging individuals to speak up. Groups are also useful for stimulating views, people will find they have strong opinions on subjects raised by others, and for generating or testing out ideas. By listening to a group in full flow, we can also learn a lot about the way in which people talk and think about important issues.

Qualitative interviews tend to be fairly long, lasting up to an hour for an individual interview and anything up to two hours for a group discussion. A large amount of rich information is generated which is usually tape-recorded and transcribed for analysis. This process of sifting and digesting the data can be time-consuming.

Since sample sizes are typically small (around 20-30 for individual interviews), random sampling of respondents for qualitative surveys is usually regarded as neither efficient nor effective. Instead, cases are selected to broaden description, contribute different insights and deepen understanding of the research topic as a whole. Such procedures come under the heading of purposive, judgmental or model based sampling.

For example, a sample of recent maternity service users may be carefully chosen to include first-time mothers as well as multigravidae, high risk as well as low risk women, those living close to services as well as those with less good access, ethnic minorities as well as majority users and so on.

Understanding basic needs and priorities

There is often little information available about what users of a service need, want or value most. There may be a clinical view about what is necessary and important, and there may be other views about what is practical or makes sense in organizational terms. We also need to know about what matters to users; this means finding ways of talking to users which allow them to communicate freely and to express themselves in terms which are most appropriate to them.

Identifying gaps or areas of weakness in broad service provision

A common concern among providers is to identify gaps or areas of weakness in the broad pattern of service provision. These may be unsuspected and there is usually an accompanying need for information which will be helpful in deciding how to fill a gap or improve an area of weakness.

'Fine-tuning' specific services

Problems often lie not so much with gaps in service as with the ways in which specific services are delivered. This is to do with matters of detail, the best ways of doing things. Again, information is needed which goes beyond identifying that there is a problem and is helpful in finding solutions. We are not asking users to tell us what to do, so much as encouraging them to tell us enough in order that we can make sensible decisions on their behalf.

Prioritising services

Most of us have to work with resources which are limited in some way and decisions have to be made about how best to use them. One element in the equation is what users value most and why, and where they would most like to see development or improvement. We may also be interested to know which areas of service they feel are less important, which needs they have which can be or are already being met in other ways.

Quantitative information may be required to tell us which are the top priorities for users as a whole. However, it may be important to know why users hold particular priorities and such information is not necessarily easily obtained through a survey. A qualitative study can help to give users the opportunity to express those reasons fully, thus deepening our understanding.

Obtaining reactions to alternative service proposals

User opinion about alternative service proposals may be helpful and again we will probably want to quantify this opinion. However, we will often want to consult users in ways which permit us to hear the reasoning behind preferences and, importantly in some cases, in ways which let us provide enough information to users about the alternatives to inform their opinions.

Measuring satisfaction with services

Perhaps the most important role for qualitative research in this area is in preparing a questionnaire that will enable us to quantify opinion. Qualitative research undertaken as a preliminary to a survey can help identify the aspects of care we need to ask about, the questions we need to ask and the language we need to use in asking them. This is the best way to ensure that we have captured relevant issues and communicated them in meaningful ways to respondents. The information from the qualitative phase will also be useful in interpreting the statistics yielded by the survey, explaining the connections between the findings from different items on the questionnaire.

Genuine involvement

Consultation with users is important in information terms, but it should also be a process which fosters genuine involvement in planning and must be seen as such.

Qualitative methods may be particularly effective in helping users to feel actively involved. They provide an opportunity for full expression of views and can easily be adapted to become settings where some exchange of information takes place.

Evaluating qualitative research

Qualitative research, like other research approaches, needs to be open to evaluation. We need to be able to make assessments about research findings and this will inevitably entail some assessment of the methods by which they were obtained.

It seems to me that there are three main sets of questions about quality in qualitative research:

- How far are the views, experiences and priorities representative of the wider population? Where samples are small and purposively selected we need to ask rigorous questions about the likely representativeness of findings, the extent to which it seems reasonable to extrapolate the findings and so on.

- How far is the information obtained and the interpretation placed on it, a 'true' or fair reflection of what users included in the study think or feel, or of how they behave?

- How reliable are the findings? Qualitative research in particular raises worries in this respect owing to the intimate relationship between the researcher and the research process at all stages.

Researchers, research commissioners and users may find the following checklist helpful when evaluating qualitative research:

1. Were appropriate sampling methods, explicitly and systematically applied?

2. Were the methods of data collection appropriate to the objectives of the research?

3. Was data-collection carried out by skilled and trained interviewers or group moderators?

4. Was the data recorded in a reliable way? (For example a tape recorder may often be more accurate than note taking)

5. Would the analytical method used stand up to external scrutiny?

Transparency in research

Qualitative researchers work in a very intimate way with their data. The process of generating information is carried out in response to an ever-evolving analysis of the situation or issues under study. The researcher should nevertheless be capable of making detached, objective sense of the subject and forming sound judgements which are not the quirky product of his or her personality or feelings. Empathy and intuition play a part but the researcher must seek constantly to ground hypotheses and ideas in data.

The process by which the researcher reaches conclusions needs to be made as transparent as possible, so that others can follow the arguments and make independent judgements about the soundness of the interpretations placed on the data. Various ways in which such transparency can be improved include:

- Use of methods during the formal analysis phase which aid systematic treatment of the data and which can be examined by others (e.g. charting)

- Clear explication of arguments or reasoning in the text of any report and appropriate use of supporting data (e.g. quotations)

- Making transcripts and tape-recordings available to research clients (suitably anonymised)

- Inviting attendance at group discussions and even interviews.

Validating qualitative research

Research is rarely carried out in an information vacuum. There will nearly always be some other source of information, be it routine, research-based (for example survey data) or locked up in the heads of experienced staff, which will provide a useful check on new research findings.

In the main, users' views should not come as a total shock to service providers or other stakeholders. You may have more or better detail, a different perspective, more solid evidence, even some completely unexpected findings, but the whole picture will usually make sense and should tally with what is already known or suspected.

Sources of information and training

Qualitative research

Walker, R. (Ed) (1985). *Applied Qualitative Research*. Gower
McCracken, G. (1988). *The Long Interview*. Sage.
Kreuger, R.A. (1988). *Focus Groups: A Practice Guide for Applied Research*.

General research methods

Sykes, W., Collins, M., Hunter, D., Popay, J., William, G. (1992). *Listening to Local Voices: A Guide to Research Methods*. Nuffield Institute for Health.
Social Research Association (1994). *Commissioning Social Research: A Good Practice Guide*. (Tel: 0171 738 6503)

Qualitative research training

Jane Ritchie, Qualitative Research Unit, Social and Community Planning Research, 35 Northampton Square, London EC1V OAX (Tel: 0171 250 1866)

Wendy Sykes
Freelance Researcher

Experiences of Listening to Women

Jo Garcia

Introduction

This paper highlights the type of useful information that can be gained from surveys of women about maternity care. These are often called 'satisfaction studies' which is unfortunate, and we should be moving away from a reliance on questions about attitudes and satisfaction to look at the issue in other ways.

Asking women what happened

Surveys of women who use the services can provide a great deal of information about key aspects of care - and for some topics are the only way to find out what you need to know. For example, the only sensible way to find out whether women are being cared for by midwives or doctors whom they have got to know is to ask them. Below is an example from the survey of women's maternity care experiences designed by Val Mason at OPCS [1,2].

At most check-ups was there someone who had got to know you and remembered you?

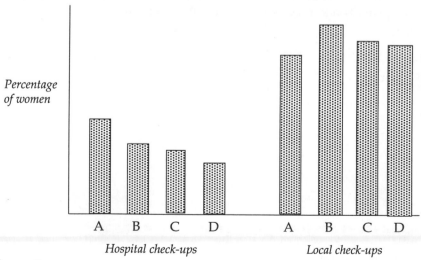

Hospital check-ups   *Local check-ups*

Figure 1

Figure 1 compares hospital antenatal clinics with locally based antenatal care. The information comes from four districts that took part in pilot studies for the questionnaire. It shows that women were more likely to say that there was someone at most check-ups who had got to know them and remembered them when describing their care at local check-ups than at the hospitals.

We can also use surveys to find out about some aspects of the clinical care that women received. There is evidence from research by Ann Cartwright (see later chapter) - who is a pioneer in this field - that the quality of such information is good. This approach has been used for aspects of care that may not be easy to study from hospital records, such as pain relief or infant feeding.

If we want to use surveys of women to assess the quality of the service, we should aim to ask women about details of their experiences and about aspects of care that they are best placed to describe. The following examples of useful questions are also drawn from the OPCS questionnaire.

Was there enough space and toys for any young children waiting at the hospital antenatal clinic?

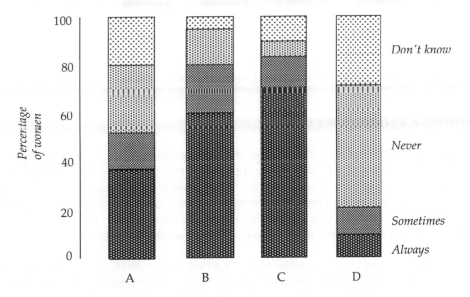

Figure 2

Answers to the question about sufficient space and toys for young children in the hospital antenatal clinic show quite big differences between the four districts that took part, and could certainly enable services to be improved. Another question with practical implications asked women whether they had the opportunity to look around the labour ward before coming in for delivery.

During this pregnancy, were you shown round the labour ward at the hospital?

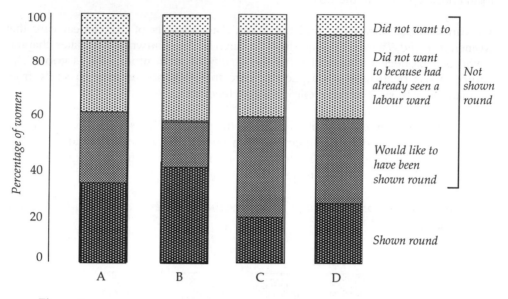

Figure 3

Again, the results show differences between the four districts.

Women's evaluations of care

If we do decide to seek women's opinions, we should do it in as specific a way as possible. The problem with focusing too much on valuations of care is that, in maternity care at least, levels of satisfaction are sometimes reported as being very high even where detailed questions reveal many problems with the care received. This is not to say that women are lying about their views, but that there is a tendency to be grateful to the midwives and doctors who give care, and a reluctance to criticise the system that has helped to produce such a good outcome for the parents.

The following example is from the survey carried out by MORI Health Research for the Expert Maternity Group, convened by the Department of Health [3]. Christine Roberts worked on this project (see Section 2). Information from their survey of women from Asian and Afro-Caribbean backgrounds can be used together with the results from the national sample. The researchers asked an evaluative question about whether women felt that they had received plenty of useful advice throughout their pregnancy.

Table 1: *'I have received plenty of useful advice throughout my pregnancy (from the different health professionals)'*

Percentage agreeing:	National	Indian	Pakistani	Bangladeshi
	66	55	54	78

Source: MORI 1993

Table 1 shows the proportions of women agreeing with the statement from the national sample and from an Indian, Pakistani, or Bangladeshi background in the ethnic minorities survey. At another point in the interview, women were also asked whether they had discussed specific items with health professionals.

	National	Indian	Pakistani	Bangladeshi
Events during labour and birth	38	15	14	6
Pain relief	50	27	15	5
Breastfeeding	40	31	23	10

Table 2: Discussed with health professionals (percent)
MORI 1993

Overall, women reported very limited discussion of these important aspects of care and it is very unlikely that over 90 per cent of women of Bangladeshi origin had no wish for information of this sort.

Conclusions

The kinds of comparison outlined in this paper need to be done for other types of question, but I feel that it does support my view that questionnaires should be as specific as possible about aspects of care that are of concern. Many of the questions that we would like to ask about care obviously contain an element of evaluation. However, I am arguing that we should avoid very general satisfaction questions and break up the care into individual components that we can ask about in detail.

Jo Garcia
Social Scientist
National Perinatal Epidemiology Unit

References
1.   Garcia, J. (1989). *Getting Consumers' Views of Maternity Care: Examples of how the OPCS Survey Manual can help*. London: Department of Health.
2.   Mason, V. (1989). *Women's Experience of Maternity Care - A Survey Manual*. London: HMSO
3.   Rudat, K., Roberts, C., Chowdhury, R. (1993). *Maternity Services: A Comparative Survey of Afro-Caribbean, Asian and White Women, Commissioned by the Expert Maternity Group*. MORI Health Research Unit, London.

Quantitative Research 2

Jenny Hewison

The starting point for this paper is that changes have been made in the provision of maternity services, that is, to the process of care. It is important to know whether those changes have made any difference to women using the service, that is to the outcome of care. Such concerns are part of a wider effectiveness agenda within the NHS.

There is currently considerable interest in measuring the outcomes of health care. Outcomes take a variety of forms: clinical, psychological and educational. Satisfaction with care is often included in this list.

My main point is that a distinction must be made between a measure and the interpretation which can be put on it. This distinction is just as important for so called 'hard' measures, such as clinical indicators, as it is for 'soft' psychological variables, such as measures of depression or social functioning, obtained by talking to women about their experiences and feelings. In each case, the main problem of interpretation is whether or not differences on the measure can be attributed to differences in care, or whether they have come about for other reasons. Using the word 'outcome' implies that the care was what made the difference. That might not be true, and casual discussion of 'outcomes' should always be treated with some caution.

Where psychological outcomes are concerned, the distinction between a measure and the interpretation which can be put on it is particularly easy to overlook. Many factors affect levels of depression, for example, besides the activities of care providers. Research in Leeds provides a useful example. Depression scores a few weeks after the birth could be partly predicted from a woman's length of hospital stay and whether her delivery had been normal, but the social background of the women was also important. The relative effects of care factors and background factors will vary in different circumstances.

This leads me to comparisons between maternity units. These are very prone to misinterpretation. Depression scores among new mothers in Tyneside are probably very high at the moment but this is much more to do with the closure of the local shipyard than it is with the care provided by the maternity services. The relative importance of different factors will vary across time and place. Unemployment and other social background factors might be most important for that place, in that year, whereas care factors might be more important somewhere else.

To reiterate an earlier point: a measure can be a good measure - sensitive, reliable, and valid - but still very difficult to interpret as an outcome. It is usually only in the special circumstances of randomised controlled trials that attributions of cause and effect can be made with confidence, and this applies to psycho-social outcomes as well as clinical ones.

This is not about accepting lower standards of care in some places that others. Rather it is about recognising that care providers can not be held responsible for poor 'outcomes', which were not in fact the result of their care.

Treating satisfaction as an outcome measure entails the same problems. 'Ceiling effects' are common with ordinary satisfaction ratings, i.e. an implausible number of people seem to be totally satisfied. There are complex connections between expectations, preferences and satisfaction. A simple example is that of waiting time. It is obvious what women prefer - who would rather wait two hours or ten minutes? But expectations have also to be considered? *'You expect to wait when you go to the doctors.'* Not surprisingly, there is conflicting evidence regarding the relationship of these variables to satisfaction.

I want to argue two separate points about satisfaction ratings - (i) to a large extent, what people rate is the way in which a given model of care is implemented, rather than the model itself. And (ii) even when they rate the success of that implementation, it is in a context of what it is reasonable to expect from those staff working in those circumstances. Caring and friendly staff who are so rushed that corners are cut are still likely to get very high satisfaction ratings: *'she did her best', 'they were so busy', 'she was only doing her job'.* It is not that you cannot access preferences about models of care: *Changing Childbirth* is a response to a ground swell of opinion and clearly stated preferences. Rather, I am arguing that once you get away from the obvious - a dislike of production lines, a preference for being treated like a human being rather than a set of reproductive organs on legs, then caution is required in interpreting ratings of satisfaction with care.

Currently, what women want is being used as a rationale for a large number of antenatal visits: *'they like regular visits and find them reassuring.'* Our data in Yorkshire suggest that women tend to like what the local service provides, which might be 14 visits, or 12 or 10. The argument is circular. Personally, I would have jumped at fewer antenatal visits if the matter had ever been discussed with me!

I will conclude by suggesting a workable approach towards the use of 'outcome measures'. I suggest that you acquaint yourselves with the main influences on the health outcomes of interest to you. You may be surprised to find that many of these influences are socio-economic. Put a list together of factors that need to be borne in mind whenever comparisons are being made, especially comparisons between maternity units. Compare like with like as far as that is possible. Always be alert to the possibility that differences in 'outcome' may be due to factors other than the care provided. Finally, be as sceptical of the results you like as you are of the results you do not like. That way, you will be going in the right direction.

Jenny Hewison
Department of Psychology and Institute of Epidemiology
and Health Services Research, University of Leeds

Using Postal Questionnaires

Ann Cartwright

Introduction
The aim of this paper is to share some of the evidence about the reliability of data from postal surveys of women having babies, and some of its snags, and to illustrate ways in which postal surveys could be useful. Such surveys can provide a wealth of information about what is happening to women, as well as data on their feelings and their reactions to the way they are treated.

Sampling
One great advantage of doing a survey of recent mothers as opposed to one of people experiencing other forms of health care, is that there is a complete and reliable register of births. This makes it possible to select a representative sample of births and using a postal approach makes it possible to have a wide geographical cover. It is also possible to use the register for local studies and to study any of the specific groups identified on the non-confidential part of the birth registration form. These include births in a particular hospital, those at home, those to mothers born in other countries or those for whom no father was identified on the birth registration form.

A reliable sampling frame of this nature means that it is not necessary to study all births to get a representative picture of what is happening. The size of the sample needed will depend on what you are interested in and how many cross-analyses you want to make. There are formulae to help calculate this. However, there is no merit in opting for a particular fraction, for example one in ten, of the population to be studied; it is the actual numbers in the sample and in the sub-groups that are important. The adequacy of the final sample and its size, however, depend on a high response rate.

Response rate
Another advantage of studying women who have had a baby is that most of them are willing to tell you about their experiences.

The response rates we had at the Institute for Social Studies in Medical Care, to postal surveys of mothers who had recently had a baby, were around 80 per cent[1]. This was after two reminders, each with a copy of the questionnaire. This compares with response rates of 88 per cent and 91 per cent to interview studies based on similar samples[2,3]. Interviews cost between twenty and fifty times as much as obtaining the data from postal surveys, however. The costs of analysis and sampling are roughly the same for both approaches if most of the answers on the postal questionnaire are precoded; that is, mothers ring the number next to the answer that applies rather than tick boxes - a procedure that does not appear to affect response rates.

However, not all mothers are equally likely to respond to postal surveys. A comparison of the information in medical records relating to mothers who did and those who did not respond to a postal questionnaire, revealed no indication of any bias related to the women's ages, their smoking habits, their previous obstetric history, including terminations, or to the tests and procedures that were carried out during pregnancy, labour and delivery[4]. The most notable bias that emerged related to the baby's health, with a low response from mothers of low birthweight babies, babies who were kept in hospital after the mother was discharged and babies admitted to special care baby units - three related events. Other significant biases related to breastfeeding and to late attendance at antenatal clinics. There was also a somewhat lower than average response from mothers not described as 'white', 'Caucasian', or 'British', and a much lower one from those whose religion was Moslem.

In another larger study comparing the data from birth registration forms for respondents and non-respondents, we found that mothers born in Asia and those with an Asian name were less likely to respond[5]. Among the non-respondents, the proportion of births for which no father was identified was relatively high. Analysis by social class as indicated by the occupation of the baby's father, gave a response rate that was higher among the middle than the working class.

The biases in relation to social class and complications associated with the baby's health also occurred in interview studies of comparable groups. Although an interviewer approach achieved a much higher response rate than the postal survey among certain ethnic minorities, the quality of the data obtained in this way, often through an interpreter, was rather dubious.

Accuracy of data

The accuracy of the data may be reviewed by comparing data obtained from a postal survey of mothers with information extracted from their medical records[6]. Good agreement between the mothers and the hospital records was observed over a wide range of events. Various reasons for inconsistencies in a few study items were identified. Mothers reported fewer terminations than in the records, probably because they wanted to forget or to conceal such events. A few mothers were apparently unaware that certain tests or procedures had been carried out, leading to a shortfall in their reports of alpha fetoprotein tests, use of pethidine and resuscitation of the baby. Ultrasound scans were more often reported by mothers than recorded in the hospital notes and a follow-up indicated that some of these had been omitted from the notes.

Another check on the accuracy of the data was a comparison of information obtained by postal questionnaire and by interview[7]. Although there was a sizeable difference in response rates, there were no major differences in the nature of responses. Reports about painful and delicate subjects were similar in both groups. If people concealed such events they did so equally often in the two situations. Topics which had been identified as emotionally laden appeared to produce a number of differences, but some in one direction, some in others. Criticisms were somewhat more likely to be reported during interviews than on postal questionnaires, particularly at open questions, which also stimulated more praise during interviews.

Postal surveys can, therefore, be reliable sources of information about many medical aspects and compare well with interview studies.

Range and nature of data

Mothers were prepared to complete quite lengthy postal questionnaires. There was no significant difference between the response rate to a questionnaire with 24 A4 pages and some 110 questions[8] and one with eight pages and 35 questions[9].

This means a wide range of topics can be covered and these can be interrelated. Women's social characteristics, obstetric history, the circumstances of the study pregnancy, labour, delivery and postnatal care, contraceptive use and family-building intentions and their preferences and views can all be cross-analysed. For example, we found that women were more likely to feel they had been treated with kindness and understanding during their labour if they were older rather than younger, white Caucasians rather than Asians or other ethnic groups, married rather than single and owner occupiers rather than council tenants[10].

Applications of this approach

This approach can be used to monitor trends in services, in their use and in women's reactions to them. It can also be used to evaluate changes in services and women's reactions to the changes. Surveys can be done at national or local level. The approach can also be used to identify particular groups for more intensive study: for example, women undergoing specific treatments, or with certain characteristics, experiences or views. It can be used as a form of audit to identify good and bad aspects of the services and unmet needs. Postal surveys are a way of listening to mothers but also of learning from them.

Ann Cartwright
Formerly Director of the Institute of Social Studies in Medical Care

References

1. Cartwright, A. (1986). 'Some Experiments with Factors that Might Affect the Response of Mothers to a Postal Questionnaire', *Statistics in Medicine*, 5, pp. 607-17.
2. Cartwright, A. (1976). *How Many Children?* London: Routledge and Kegan Paul.
3. Cartwright, A. (1979). T*he Dignity of Labour?* London: Tavistock.
4. Cartwright, A. (1986). 'Who Responds to Postal Questionnaires?', *Journal of Epidemiology and Community Health*, 40, pp.267-73.
5. See 4.
6. See 4.
7. Cartwright, A. (1988). 'Interviews or Postal Questionnaires? Comparisons of Data about Women's Experience with Maternity Services', *The Millbank Quarterly*, 66, pp.172-89.
8. See 1.
9. see 1.
10. See 4

Experiences of Listening to Women: The Importance of Ethno-Centric Research

Carole Baxter

Introduction

Whilst there has been an increase in consumer involvement in the planning and development of services, the views of some users have been inadequately or poorly represented. Despite an increasing recognition that all users have the right to give their views about a particular service, there is considerable uncertainty about the appropriate methods for ensuring that these views are heard.

There is a need for a strategy which recognises the diverse nature of the population and which is effective in canvassing the views of those sections who have experiences, priorities and expectations which differ from the majority population.

Most investigations into the views of women using the maternity services ignore the perspective of black and ethnic minority women. They lack appropriate methods of obtaining the views of different groups of women. It is important to recognise and treat race and ethnicity as a serious area in need of investigation.

There is a definitional problem over what 'black' and 'ethnic minority' mean for some people. The 1991 Census provided a list of categories which included around six per cent of the UK population, of whom approximately half were women.

Race and ethnicity in research methods

The diverse nature of the black and ethnic minority population should be recognised; for instance, social and economic status differ widely. It is possible to focus work on those who are most likely to experience discrimination, such as poor people and those who do not speak English. Deprivation is a primary contributor to poor health status and lack of access to services.

The following issues need to be considered.

* Some people are not used to being asked their views
* Husbands tend to answer, especially for those women who do not speak English
* There may be a fear of being critical.
* Trust will need to be developed
* Confidentiality is an area of concern for most women

What is being investigated?

In addition to quantitative data, experience, views, attitudes and beliefs should all be considered. The latter particularly are often problem areas in terms of recognition by the health service. Where black and ethnic minority women are consulted there is too often a cultural rather that an anti-racist approach, with too little attention given to issues of racism and discrimination. On the other hand, users are rarely confident enough to tell researchers about their experience of racism. Studies have identified that approximately ten per cent of users mention racism; however, a larger group experience attitudes which are racist but do not label them as such.

Finally, the experiences of black and ethnic minority women are often contrasted with those of white women. Similarities of experience are not ordinarily looked for.

Methodology

The diverse nature of Britain's black and ethnic minority population must be recognised. When collecting data, recognised classifications (OPCS, Commisssion for Racial Equality and DoH) should be used to identify ethnic origin.

A combination of quantitative and qualitative methods is needed to make research or consultation credible. These may include:

- Focus groups
- Interviews
- Diary keeping, possibly using a tape recorder
- Comparative studies of interethnic and white families
- Surveys
- Rapid participative research - feeding results back rapidly to improve service
- Use of same race, bilingual workers may be preferable
- Translation should be local - dialects may be different between areas
- Advocates can help where women feel disempowered and there is a language barrier.

Who is going to do the research?

Research is not objective or sterile in the way it is presented. Black researchers have an important role to play, and not just in the collection of data. It is crucial that black workers are involved in the design and planning of the investigation. They are more likely to have credibility with the community being researched because of unequal power relationships which exist between black and white people in our society. Black researchers are also more likely to have the same experience as the group they are studying, such as experiencing racism. Without that kind of perception, the issue may not be openly discussed.

Reported views may be passed through a white cultural filter if a black researcher is not used. There is also the lack of an insider perception, whereas black researchers have generally developed an understanding of both minority and majoprity cultures. Skills can be shared with white researchers.

The researcher can explain their interest to participants, such as 'we know there are problems; our babies are dying more than white babies', to demonstrate why they are concerned and listening.

Research management

It is important for black and ethnic minority groups to be involved with the research management. The black voluntary sector is often a source of appropriate researchers. They have access to the community and skills to carry out the research. If relationships are developed at an early stage, issues of funding, publication and ownership of results can be worked through to ensure that the research is responsive to the needs of women and action will be taken on the results. One such organization actively involved is Manchester Action Committee on Healthcare for Ethnic Minorities. (MACHEM). This is a voluntary organization made up of groups and individuals primarily from black and ethnic minority communities.

Health professionals doing their own research must be aware of the obligation to be honest in reporting their results, however unpopular they may be. Whether it is possible to implement any changes as a result of findings should be considered before initiating the research. This includes student research projects.

Ethics

Ethics committees need to be aware of the priority to feed back results of the research to those involved. Expertise to assess the results of studies by those on these committees should be enhanced.

The use of inner city poor in public health research, depriving women of a service in order to identify differences, is one reason why the involvement of ethics committees is essential. However, the experience within such committees to assess studies for their soundness in terms of race relations is thin on the ground.

Carole Baxter
Senior Lecturer, University of Central Lancashire, Chair of
Manchester Action Committee on Health Care for Ethnic Minorities.
Consultant, Black and Ethnic Minority Groups, Changing Childbirth Teams

References:
1.   Office of Population Censuses and Surveys (1991). *Census Data Local Base Studies.* OPCS.

An Overview of Three Research Methodologies - Benefits and Drawbacks

Margaret Reid

Involving consumers

Research in the maternity services should involve consumers at as many stages as possible. This is not always as easy as it might sound. When planning and designing a study it is important to ascertain what the key issues for consumers are. Pilot studies are one way that women can add to a pre-decided questionnaire schedule.

Writing up and presentation of the research are two stages at which it is sometimes more difficult to involve consumers; time scales may not allow for draft reports to be circulated to those who responded. At the very least, research results should be fed back to consumer groups, via a maternity services liaison committee, consumer groups such as NCT, or a community health council. If necessary, they should be given the opportunity for indirect feedback to the research funders.

When to research mothers experiences

One much debated point is when to carry out the research. Before pregnancy might be ideal for some studies, but it is virtually impossible to find a group of women who may become pregnant in the next weeks or months. Sometimes women are asked 'If you were pregnant, what would you choose...?. This method of asking women hypothetically has its drawbacks, as people do not always end up doing what they had said they might.

Many studies are carried out antenatally, and there may be good reason to do this. However, some women may feel diffident about reporting complaints about the service, and so rather bald questionnaires looking for levels of consumer satisfaction may receive bland responses of 'very satisfied'; women may feel vulnerable, grateful to the staff and in no mood for reflection about the situation they are in. If, on the other hand, the questionnaire takes a rather different approach and divides the major questions into issues which women feel that they can comment on without detriment to their care, a more illuminating response is likely.

It is tempting to 'move in' once the baby has been born and to ask the 'captive population' of mothers in hospital about their maternity care. The sampling and interviewing may be easy; large hospitals have considerable numbers of mothers of whom many appear to be willing to talk about their experiences. However, research has indicated that a 'halo' effect operates immediately after the birth, and mothers who report considerable satisfaction with everything may, in a few weeks time start to voice some concerns. Practically, too, early discharge means that many women leave hospital within the first three days of giving birth, so that the 'captive population' of the past may be less in evidence today.

There is now a general consensus that the optimum time to ask women about their maternity care, antenatal and postnatal, is a few weeks after the birth. Research should never be too intrusive, and turning up on the doorstep immediately the baby is home has not proved very convenient for many mothers. A few weeks later may be both kinder and may achieve a more considered picture of what the mother experienced. She will have had time to reflect, to remember the good and the less good parts of the experience, and be able to help the research study with these reflections.

However, a few researchers have gone further and returned to the families some months after the birth. What they found was that the 'halo' that existed in the early days had disappeared and that women could be more critical of their care at this time than they were previously.

It is difficult to argue which approach gives the 'truest' picture. It is important simply to recognise the possible biases of timing.

Fathers too!

It is also important to add here that the majority of studies have focused upon the women's experiences, while those of the father are neglected. Many women go into the experience as a couple and go through it as a couple. Feelings and beliefs about maternity care are arrived at through discussion with the partner and although the woman alone undergoes the unique experience of giving birth, the father's views and experiences are not as irrelevant as the dearth of research would suggest.

Who should carry out the research?

Who should carry out the study? Ideally, all research should be carried out by independent trained researchers, whether they are based in a research unit, a university, are freelance researchers or whatever. Researchers have the necessary experience to make the right decisions about the methods appropriate to the study and about carrying out the analysis and writing the report.

Be aware of the biases contained within who approaches the consumer, since this may influence the research findings. Long experience has indicated that if approached by a member of staff, even a junior female member of staff, then many women tend to give more favourable responses.

Ethics

How much do the women know about the study and how much should they know? Women should be presented with a clear statement about the research and its intention. Each woman should be given time to think about her possible involvement. Becoming involved in a research study can change people; perhaps this is the first time they have stopped to think about aspects of their experience, or perhaps the study has forced them to re-think something they had previously chosen to forget. Poorly carried out research, or research which upsets the consumer is unfair as well as damaging.

Research methodologies: quantitative methods

Questionnaires are widely used for collecting factual and attitudinal information. They can be composed of 'closed choice' questions where the subject has to fit her response into a range of options, or they can allow some input from the subject who writes in her answers to 'open-ended' questions. Devising a questionnaire is very difficult as you have to know what the possible answers might be before you start. You can avoid this by offering more open-ended questions but one of the beauties of a questionnaire study is that it can be relatively easily analysed, and open-ended questions make this more difficult. Questionnaire studies provide the majority of data in the form of numbers (and tables) which is still attractive to many funders.

Benefits:
- Relatively quick/large sample/standardised
- Variety of ways of administering (e.g. sent by mail, person to person)
- Anonymous - respondent may express views more confidently
- Quick analysis can give rapid feedback
- Results immediately 'accessible' (e.g. through tables etc.)

Drawbacks:
- Lack of flexibility
- Results about 'what' women think not 'why'
- Not women's own words
- Sample size could be a problem (need reasonably large numbers)
- Need to know key issues before start

Interviews and focus groups are qualitative methods that will produce a rather different output, mainly words rather than numbers. You are finding out about what people think about their world and the experience is interpreted through their words. Qualitative methods can be explanatory - WHY something is happening rather than what is happening.

Research methodologies: interviews

Interviews are particularly suited to studying beliefs, feelings, opinions, views, experiences, things that are less easy to say 'yes' and 'no' to. They are face-to-face discussions in which the researcher has a number of questions which are put to the interviewee who then responds in his or her own words. They can be used to explore a field or, conversely, to do an in-depth study once key issues have been identified. They are also useful if you have people for whom English is not their first language although obviously you need interpreters.

Benefits:
- Usually good response rate
- Flexibility, you can incorporate changes if necessary
- Uses subjects own words, no interpretation necessary

- Provides very rich data, can help understand how subjects feel
- Non-verbal data can be important

Drawbacks:
- Time consuming to carry out interviews and often expensive
- Time-consuming to analyse
- Small sample numbers, some funders may not like this
- Greater influence of researcher, potential for bias unless researchers trained
- Might be a topic about which subject has not much to say

Research methodologies: focus groups

Focus groups are informal groups brought together to discuss the research topic. They can offer a quick overview of the range of opinions people hold about a certain topic. While pure sampling may be difficult, groups can be organized to maximise the possible range of views (e.g. by making sure that different age groups are represented, or by separately organising groups of older women or teenage girls, first time mothers/ second or more mothers etc.). Focus groups should be small 4 or 6-10 is about right and they should not last too long, 1-2 hours is often enough.

The end product of focus groups will be words, not numbers; their strength is the overall range of views which can be relatively quickly collected.

Benefits:
- Can be carried out quite quickly and cheaply
- Explicit discussion on topic of research
- 'Group' processes can draw out individuals
- Can get views of a range of people
- 'Story telling' quality as illustration/naturalistic vocabulary on topic
- Less impact of researcher as others take over questioning
- Less preparation

Drawbacks:
- Artificial', depends on sampling as to how artificial
- Dominant individuals can suppress others
- Limited to studying verbal behaviour
- Interaction only within discussion groups
- Created and managed by researcher
- Bias towards the articulate individual
- Group dynamic may reduce limit the range of views expressed

Many researchers now mix methods, combining, for example, focus groups to alert the researcher to the key issues for the women and then perhaps carrying out a questionnaire study with a larger sample. This kind of mix and match approach is useful, although dividing a study into several stages inevitably takes longer.

Margaret Reid
Senior Lecturer
Department of Public Health, Glasgow University

A Case Study of Research in Action: The Audit Commission

Jocelyn Cornwall

Introduction

This short paper is based on the Audit Commission's research into communication between acute hospitals and patients, published in 1993. The data was collected in 16 hospitals in England and Wales in 1992.

Some of the questions we wanted to answer in the research were:

- Do the people providing the service know what patients think of the service
- How do they find out patients' view
- If there is a variety of methods is there one best method? Are some more appropriate or more successful than others?

This paper has two inter-linked themes which are the management of feedback from patients and procedural and practical questions about standards of research and expertise.

Methodologies

The methods hospitals have available to them for obtaining feedback can be divided into 'passive' and 'active' methods:

- 'Passive' methods. The hospital provides the name and address of someone to whom patients and others may tell their views (formally or informally), but does not take any other action. Examples: complaints, thank you letters and suggestion boxes.

- 'Active' methods. These include a wide variety of different approaches that hospitals take to seek out the views of patients. Examples: questionnaire based surveys; interview based surveys, which can be face to face or conducted on the 'phone; the 'mystery patient' technique; consulting local voluntary organizations and the Community Health Council; focus groups; patient participation groups and advisory panels.

Problems

We found a number of common problems in the research that is actively undertaken in hospitals into patients' views. These include research which:

- Is initiated either by enthusiasts or as part of a student project. As a result it is often piecemeal and fragmented. Some wards and departments have a great deal of research activity going on, and the patients are consulted again and again, whilst in others, there is very little or no research at all. Research studies are also rarely repeated or followed up year on year, so that it is not possible to explore trends, or to find out if something that was a problem at one time has or has not been resolved.

- Focuses on aspects of the hospital that do not feel very significant or important to patients. Questionnaire based surveys are the preferred methods of research in the majority of cases, and although it is routine to ask questions about hotel aspects of care, car parking, directions and travel, it is much less common to find questions about aspects of care that other sources tell us matter more to patients, such as the communication they have with the health professionals looking after them, or their views on the humanity and dignity of the care offered.

- Starts without any kind of literature review or investigation of previous research in the same area. There is a fairly continuous process of going over and over the same ground which often results from previous research not having been acted upon.

- Is done to a rather poor standard. Examples include: poorly designed and laid out questionnaires; questionnaires in print that is too small (less than 12 point) for people with visual impairments to read easily; questions poorly phrased so that the answers are ambiguous; interviews conducted by people without any training in interviewing techniques; study samples selected in such a way that is impossible to do any kind of testing for statistical significance; poor presentation of results and poor report writing skills.

- Is not part of an overall plan for the department or ward, and is done without any kind of advance commitment to take action on the results.

- Is completed without either the staff or the patients who take part in the research receiving feedback on the results.

Overcoming the problems

The solutions to the poor standard of research lie with management. The management function here is to lead the work, in the sense of making sure that it is part of an overall programme or strategy for quality assurance and improvements in services to patients, and that it commands the resources that are necessary for it to be done properly.

Once it is embedded in a strategic programme, it becomes possible to look at questions of resource, such as: who should do the work; what kind of expertise is required; can it be done in-house, or is there a need to get outside help?

It is crucial to ask in advance whether the purpose of the research is: to find out answers to questions that are entirely new or to measure patients' perceptions in a field where their views are already well known. If the purpose is to enter new territory altogether, to find out what patients think in an area where the research has very little idea of the range of patients' views, it is sensible to adopt a qualitative method of research. If it is to gauge how much or how little patients share a view that is already fairly well known, then it is more appropriate to use a quantitative research method. Both have their place.

Here, it is important to think through a number of questions in advance of undertaking the work, including:

- What kind of analysis is appropriate;
- Who will do the analysis;
- Do they have sufficient time and expertise to do it properly;
- Which is the best method of presenting the findings?

Conclusions

Only management commitment to the work can make it possible to develop higher standards in the conduct of the research. It also makes it more likely that:

- Previous work in the same area will be taken into account;
- There will be an advance commitment to take action on the findings;
- The questions the research is intended to answer will be specified more carefully, which means that the answers, in turn, are more likely to be useful.

Jocelyn Cornwall
Assistant Director
Health Studies Directorate, Audit Commission

A Case Study of Research in Action: The Swindon Consumer Involvement Project

Susan Clarke & Annie Naji

'When those who are used to speaking out learn to listen, and those who are used to listening learn to speak out, then we'll have real change.' [1]

Introduction

This chapter introduces the Consumer Involvement Project, explains briefly its approach to consumer involvement and what can be learnt about putting research methods into practice.

The Consumer Involvement Project was set up as a three year, fixed term, action research project funded by the Gatsby Charitable Foundation. Its main aim of which was to encourage Swindon Health Authority to improve its responsiveness to consumers.

Whilst many important lessons were learnt during the Project's life, one of the most important and pertinent was that carefully applied and selected methods do not necessarily mean good consumer involvement.

Obviously good consumer involvement requires appropriate methods but it is easy to underestimate the importance of the factors which influence the selection of appropriate methods and the importance of organizational change and development.

The Project itself was not about consulting any particular groups of users, nor was it committed to any particular method. Rather, it was set up to improve the involvement of all consumers in the planning and delivery of health care. So it was in part about working with Swindon Health Authority to raise awareness and change the internal culture of the organization.

The Project was set up with a fairly broad framework within which to develop its work. The key tenet to our approach was that there are five essential features of consumerism, namely:

Access:　　　　What services are offered to whom?
　　　　　　　　　How easy are they to use?
　　　　　　　　　Where are they?

Choice: Can consumers influence the provision of services?
Are users' interests considered?
Are their views part of the service-monitoring procedures?

Information: Are consumers fully informed about services?
Do providers seek out, and react to, information from users?

Redress: Do clear and efficient complaint/feedback procedures exist?
Are they well publicised?
Is consumer feedback used to inform changes in practice?

Representation: Are users' views sought and made known wherever decisions
are made?
Are voluntary organizations consulted?
Is there a system of advocacy in place?

We took the view that by tackling the implications of each of these features, purchasers and providers can develop a useful framework for user involvement. In addition, we maintained that consumer involvement can, and should, take place at three levels:

- The individual level
- The collective level
- Through representation

The Project also argued that good consumer involvement would require more than just working with direct users of services. Marilyn Taylor[2] offers a useful categorisation of the different user groups which we used to inform our thinking.

- **Direct users:**   People actually using a service (patients or clients)
- **Indirect users:**   including carers, partners or parents
- **Excluded users:**   People who need services but fail to use them
- **Potential users:**   People who may need services in the future
- **Proxy users:**   For example voluntary organizations, care managers, GPs, the public

The Project had five workers, none of whom had backgrounds in the NHS. We worked in both purchaser and provider settings and, over the three years that the Project ran, completed many different pieces of work. The Project used a wide range of methods but always emphasised the consumer perspective.

In all of the work, our approach was to work with staff and not simply to collect views ourselves. This was because we wanted to ensure that staff were able to continue the work after the Project ended.

The emphasis was on building on-going relationships between the Authority and consumers, or the 'wider public'. Not only did the Authority have to be prepared to change its perspective, but also the public needed to be encouraged to give its views.

As a Project we also had to compromise and found ourselves on occasion using methods, like a survey, in a not entirely appropriate situation, in order to demonstrate the potential for consumer involvement and to encourage staff to dip their toes into what often appears to be very murky water.

Carefully applied methods do not necessarily mean good consumer involvement will naturally result. In our experience it has been shown that good consumer involvement requires organizational change and development to go hand in hand with the implementation of the various research methods. Practical research can not be effective in a policy vacuum.

So, what does organizational change and development mean?

Be clear about why you are working with consumers

One of the greatest challenges facing health authorities who want to work towards effective consumer involvement is to recognise the need, to be clear about why they want to involve consumers. Thinking carefully about some of the many good reasons for involving consumers can provide a good impetus for getting the 'how' of consumer involvement right.

Be flexible and willing to demonstrate change

Working with consumers frequently requires health authorities, to do things differently and mistakes are bound to be made, so it is important that strategies are flexible enough to encompass necessary changes. Likewise, services need to be flexible - organizations must be prepared to demonstrate some action, however small, very fast, otherwise people get fed up with what they see as all talk and no action. Needless to say, for speedy responses to requests for change or action it is important to have a clear mechanism for feeding issues into the decision making process.

Empowering staff

Staff are, in the current climate, feeling vulnerable - particularly in the light of what seems to be non-stop organizational reform. Working with consumers in partnership can challenge the legitimacy, effectiveness and status of health professionals and managers whose training often teaches them to know the answers; it does not equip them to learn from the community and actively seek views. We, that is health care professionals, need to move from being the health expert to engaging in an equal partnership with consumers.

It is important, then, to ensure that staff are empowered by their organization to work with communities and consumers. Equally essential is that staff are genuinely given enough time to get out there and engage with people, in addition to the time set aside to implement the chosen method. What people have to say in informal discussions may well have a significant effect on how you implement your method or even which method you use.

Go beyond the individual user

There are many people whose views may be radically different to those of the people who actually use services, but these views are nonetheless vitally important to the future development of services which meet everybody's needs. So when you are selecting a method it is important to think beyond those which will only access the views of direct users and to consider other user groups including voluntary organizations.

Conclusions

We have learnt that successfully selecting and implementing your method of consulting with users is important, but that it is only a means to an end. Equally important is a full understanding of the issues which will determine the eventual success of the research in effecting change - not least of which, as we have painfully discovered, is organizational change and development.

Susan Clarke and Annie Clarke
Formerly researchers,
Swindon Consumer Involvement Project

References
1.   Porter, S. (1993). Community Health Action, Issue 28 Summer.
2.   Taylor, M., Hayes, L., Lart, R., Means, R. (1992). 'User empowerment in community care: unravelling the issues', School of Advanced Urban Studies, Bristol.

Researching the Needs of Disabled Parents: 1

Jo O'Farrell

Introduction

ParentAbility is a National Childbirth Trust network supporting pregnancy and parenthood for disabled parents. Through its work, it is in regular contact with over 450 disabled parents and parents-to-be and is frequently consulted by a wide variety of organizations, including purchasers and providers of maternity services, seeking the views of disabled people.

Working with disabled users of services

Disabled people are as diverse in their views and needs as people without disabilities. A range of methods of consultation will, therefore, be appropriate. Certain common rules apply, however, and if the maternity services are really committed to genuine consultation with disabled users, we recommend the following key points be incorporated into the process.

- Go to where disabled people are; do not expect them to come to you. Use the disability information services, Centres for Integrated/Independent Living and other networks to make contact with disabled users.

- Make your consultation papers accessible. Produce them in appropriate formats such as large print, Braille, tape or video film. Use signs and graphics, Makaton and the languages of the local community. Use simple, plain language that is free of jargon.

- Make your consultation meetings accessible. Provide transport, child care, facilitators and expenses to cover the costs of attending. Make sure the venue is fully accessible and that the meeting is at a reasonable time for parents of young children. Allow sufficient time for disabled people to take rest and comfort breaks and do not make meetings too long. Sessions should be taped and interpreted when required.

- Be creative in the ways you consult. Attend regular meetings of disability groups, use the telephone and telephone-networking, invite written or taped responses or offer personal interviews, and use computer networks.

- Allow sufficient time for people to respond. Disabled users may need more time to consult, discuss and reply. Time scales are usually much too tight.

- Fund the costs of consultation. Most voluntary networks operate on a shoe-string and it costs them money to send out papers, make calls and arrange meetings. Offer administrative facilities to help with this.

- Make sure that everyone who contributes gets information about the results of the consultation. Disabled people must feel that their effort is worthwhile and that their views will be listened to, if they are to put their time, energy and resources into consultation.

- Buy a copy of *Involving Disabled People in Community Care Planning* by Catherine Bewly and Caroline Glendinning, published by the University of Manchester Press in 1994. This is a report of a research project which investigated, evaluated and examined the ways in which disabled people have been, and can be, effectively involved in service planning. (See Caroline Glendinning's paper in this Section).

Jo O'Farrell
Honorary Secretary
NCT Parentability

Researching the Needs of Disabled Parents: 2

Caroline Glendinning

Introduction

This paper records the experience of consulting disabled users of community care services and suggests that these principles could be applied to consulting disabled users of maternity services.

Under the 1990 NHS and Community Care Act, local authorities are required annually to produce plans of their community care services. The first community care plans were published in April 1992, a year before the main community care changes. The preparation of these plans is to be 'marked by collaboration and joint working with, and by the involvement of, through consultation, service users'. However, no guidelines have been issued on *how* this consultation is to be carried out.

The Joseph Rowntree Foundation funded a two year project to evaluate the effectiveness of different methods of consultation and to identify the hidden barriers experienced by disabled people in getting their voices heard. It placed a special focus on older people, black people, people with learning and sensory disabilities and people whose first language is not English. The project involved an in-depth study of five local areas, and talking to a wide range of organizations both of and for disabled people.

Consultation through representation

The first year of 'consultation' was embedded in widespread publicity about the forthcoming community care changes. As community care planning became more of an annual routine, there was an increasing tendency to embed consultation in the structures and processes of drawing up plans, by inviting representatives onto planning teams and working parties. This raises a number of issues.

WHO SELECTS THE REPRESENTATIVES?
It is not sufficient for statutory officers to hand pick representatives:

> *They prefer the individual users because they're much easier to handle and manipulate and they can hand pick them. So, we have a whole group of hand-picked users who go to user meetings - hand picked by social services - and then we're told that social services is consulting with users.* (Paid worker from an organization of disabled people)

Sometimes voluntary organizations are asked to nominate a 'representative' - but representative of whom? Of the organization's own members, of all disabled service users or of all disabled people?

TIME TO CONSULT

Schedules of meetings must allow time for representatives to discuss proposals with their constituent organizations.

WHO REPRESENTS WHOM?

Representation should not be by disabled officers:

> *With regard to consultation with people with physical disabilities, it should be noted that the social services officer who chaired the group in 1990/91 and 1991/1992 was himself disabled, and he represented consumer views admirably.* (Health authority manager)

Nor should it be by carers, especially of learning disabled people:

> *Good practice is that you aren't asking parents and carers for their views on their son or daughter; you're actually asking them what their own needs are. I think that if the local authority doesn't have that difference clear in its own mind, there is a terrible confusion.* (Mencap development worker)

Some statutory officers express anxiety about organizations of disabled people - are they really 'representative'?

> *This [representativeness issue] is a classic social services way of having a go at us. Social services are quite good with any organization they find threatening; they find ways to discredit them. It's classic social services speak - I've heard it so many times, either directly or indirectly. In fact we're in touch with a damn sight more local organizations than they are, is the answer to that one.* (Paid worker from an organization of disabled people)

CONFIDENCE TO PARTICIPATE

A number of study participants argued that at least two user representatives should be allowed at any meeting, as a single user representative can easily feel intimidated by the language, jargon or formal procedures at meetings or by a lack of background information.

Practical issues

There are important issues to be considered whatever specific method of consultation is used.

LANGUAGE AND FORMAT

Community care planning processes place a heavy reliance on written English, with a liberal sprinkling of jargon. Material must be produced in a variety of formats:

- Ethnic minority languages
- Welsh
- BSL/Makaton
- Braille
- Tape

Some black people may not be able to read the language they speak because of illiteracy or visual impairment:

> *When you're trying to do consultation with the Asian community, you do need to have an Asian worker, you do need to have somebody to do the actual work outside, to knock on people's doors. That's the only way.* (Asian resource centre co-ordinator)

THE COSTS OF CONSULTATION

Consultation can be expensive, both for individuals and organizations:

> *There is no recognition of the fact that to get people to go to meetings involves time, phone calls, their travel costs which the organization often has to pay, if they have child care, all that sort of business.* (Paid worker from an organization of disabled people)

Costs associated with consultation need to be recognised and reimbursed.

ACCESS AND PARTICIPATION

Encouraging and enabling disabled people to take part means considering:

- Physical access   do lifts accommodate wheelchairs?
- Communication   BSL/loop systems/making sure that people can lip-read
- Timing   don't start too early so that participants can take advantage of cheap fares
- Duration   regular comfort breaks and deadlines for finishing meetings
- Location   go to users rather than expecting them to come to you.

PROVIDING BACKGROUND INFORMATION AND ENGAGING IN COMMUNITY DEVELOPMENT
Consultation cannot take place 'cold'. People need background information to understand the issues and questions on which they are being consulted. In some communities this may be better transmitted face to face rather than in written form.

EXPECTATIONS, GOALS AND CHANGE
Be clear and realistic about the goals of consultation and how it relates to decision-making and change. If disabled service users are encouraged to expect change to follow consultation and do not see it happening, they will quickly become disillusioned. Consultation must be part of a genuine commitment to act on the views expressed by users of services.

> *...There are constitutions drawn up but they tend to say that planning groups will meet six times a year rather than what they'll do when they've met. It doesn't clearly define what their power is and what it isn't and within the group who's got it....If [a vote] is carried, what does it change: has that just decided planning group policy or has it actually changed budgets?* (District health authority assistant director)

Caroline Glendinning
Formerly Department of Social Policy
University of Manchester

Researching the Needs of Families with Sick Babies

Jenny White

Introduction

Consultation can often be an important part of an individual's care as well as an assessment of a service as a whole. In the context of neonatal care in the community, the whole family's needs and wishes must be recognised, respected and acted upon. This paper identifies five stages of care which form a continual process of learning and development: identifying need; responding; action; reviewing achievement; and evaluation, all of which involve listening carefully to service users.

Identifying need

A family's need for community support is assessed by talking to the parents, asking questions and listening so that they may share their feelings and experiences. Some people are extremely anxious about taking their new baby home, particularly if they have had problems with a previous baby. They often refer to feeling 'anxious', 'totally isolated', 'lonely', 'frightened', 'lacking support', 'unable to sleep', 'so worried and I spent most of the time crying' or 'inadequate and a failure'.

Responding to need

The aim of a community support service is to develop nursing care for babies that, by supporting their families, allows them to remain at home. Such a service requires the identification of suitably qualified staff, funding, resources, training and an efficient system of communication between all parties.

Action

The community support service establishes a link between hospital and home by liaising with health visitors, GPs, midwives, health service managers, hospital staff, parents and the support services. GP fund-holders, in particular, have been made aware of what the service offers and its advantages. The limits of the service must also be identified and boundaries set. Home Care Services provide many dimensions of care.

- Nursing care - including drug administration, feeding, application of dressings, oxygen administration, monitoring, post-operative care and care associated with congenital abnormalities and life-threatening illnesses

- Psychological care - including supportive visits to parents and their families who are under stress, a counselling service

- Continuous care - liaison with ward and community staff and other health care professionals to ensure good continuity of care for families

- Consistent care - maintenance of clear and precise records of all care, support and advice given, ensuring good communication between all parties

Reviewing achievement

Progress is reviewed through regular team meetings, client satisfaction assessments, monitoring developments and measuring quality outcomes. The aim of such review is to expand the Home Care Service so that hospital admissions and length of stay are kept to a minimum and the cost of neonatal care is reduced.

Cases which illustrate our work include that of a boy who, though still oxygen-dependent at three years old, had been able to leave hospital aged five months. Without the Home Care Service supporting his family he would still be hospitalised. In another, a six month old baby with multiple problems was able to be cared for at home before she died. This meant a great deal to her family who are left with many special memories.

Evaluation

Following review of what the service has achieved, the processes of care may be amended as necessary, implementing improvements and extending the service as further needs and developments are identified. These might include:

- More continuing care and support for families following a stillbirth
- Respite care
- Regular infant resuscitation classes
- Purchase of equipment to provide phototherapy treatment at home
- Support, counselling and advice prior to birth, now made possible as a result of improvements in the antenatal detection of problems.

Evaluating the service feeds into the identification of need thus completing the circular process of care.

Jenny White
Neonatal Community Nurse Specialist
Queen Elizabeth II Hospital
Welwyn Garden City

Researching the Needs of Women from Minority Communities

Robina Khawaja

Introduction

Clearly one of the major challenges in consulting users is to communicate effectively with non-English speakers. Often empowerment is a prerequisite stage before consultation. This paper describes on approach to empowering women.

This session began in Urdu. Most of the audience did not understand and when asked how they felt, someone commented 'It serves us right!'

I explained that I wanted them to understand a little of how it feels when the speaker is fluent and the listener is not. Body language and tone of voice contribute to our understanding, even when the words do not mean anything, but when verbal communication is not effective, the listener may feel anger or worry and will in time lose interest and may even stop listening.

Effective communication

Within the health care setting, there are three broadly different types of workers whose remit revolves around effective communication on behalf of either professionals or clients, or both. The roles and responsibilities of interpreters, language support workers and advocates are summarised below.

Interpreters

An interpreter is called on behalf of a professional to provide an oral translation of one language into another, usually for a fee. It is important to note that no other interaction should take place.

Language Support Workers (LSW) (also known as linkworkers)

Professionals also instigate the services of LSWs. LSWs contribute awareness of cultural issues and of religious values in addition to their language skills. They must speak the dialect of the target community, not just the language. LSWs are usually employed directly by the health care organization in which they work.

Advocates

(Editors' note - The advocacy service in Leeds is independent of the health service, being provided by voluntary organizations and the local council.) Advocacy is usually a free service, initiated by the client not the professional. Advocates offer awareness of culture and religious values and speak the local community dialect, but they are also able to give their clients information, ask questions on their behalf and aim to empower them and service their needs rather than those of the professionals.

Misunderstandings and antipathy from professionals sometimes arise because of confusion between advocacy and interpreting. Advocates always act on behalf of their clients first. They aim to empower their clients by ensuring that they have full access to services and knowledge of what is available and being offered. Within this role, an advocate may question a professional on behalf of her client, and it is this aspect of the advocate's work which may be seen as threatening or time-consuming. Advocacy should not be seen as any more time-consuming than responding to the needs of any other client who wants more information. When a professional feels uncomfortable in such a situation, the professional and advocate should clarify the role each is playing and the expectations each has of the session. If these issues are addressed beforehand, misunderstandings should be avoided.

A health professional may be refused an advocate when the client has not been informed. The advocate is there on behalf of the client, something which is incompatible with the client being unaware that advocacy is taking place. Advocacy organizations will expect the initiative to come from the client and will check this by contacting them directly. Health professionals have a tendency to ask for an advocate only when a problem has arisen and they need someone to interpret for them. Such conflicts can be avoided only if an organization directly employs LSWs trained to meet its needs and those of patients, or by allowing advocacy to operate properly.

The role of the professional

Sensitivity to cultural issues and respect for religious values will enhance effective communication. However, health professionals may occasionally feel unable to understand certain practices, in which case, the only response is to accept that this is what the client wants and to respect their decision.

Each client is an individual; judgements based on stereotypes and previous bad experiences with clients from a similar background are not helpful. Professionals should address communication difficulties directly, and use sensitive questions and effective visual material to improve communication.

Leeds Family Health - 1994 Initiatives

The Leeds Family Health Services Authority (FHSA) undertook research in 1992 into the maternity services needs and experiences of ethnic minority women locally. I was appointed in September 1994 to help address the needs of Asian women as highlighted by the research. Some other recent initiatives are outlined below.

Haamla classes

Parentcraft classes are available for English-speaking women but are not accessible to those with other language needs. 'Haamla' (Urdu for 'pregnant woman') classes are being developed as an alternative.

The classes are held in the community to give easy access for women. A midwife and an advocate attend and there is a crèche. The first class, in the Harehills Community Centre, aims to provide appropriate care, information and support for Asian women. Once these classes have been established, others will be developed at different venues within Leeds.

Community links

Good links within the community are being forged by outreach work, including through my post. The support of other workers already effectively involved locally is being won. This is important for the provision of appropriate services but particularly if we are to encourage minority group representation at planning and senior management levels within our organizations.

Advocacy services and GP surgeries

The FHSA has established links with the advocacy services so that when targeting primary health care providers on behalf of the minority ethnic communities, the support of advocates is available. GPs are being encouraged to assess the effectiveness of their services to clients whose first language is not English. They are also being encouraged to work with advocates willing to support their clients in visits to the GP. Advocacy is about to begin within selected surgeries in ChapelTown and Harehills. The aim is to offer support eventually to all surgeries interested in taking part. GPs have identified language and improved understanding of community and hospital services as areas in which women need support, and advocacy is one way in which we can act on these needs.

Robina Khawaja
Primary Health Care, Development Worker
(Maternity services), Leeds Family Health Services Authority

Maintaining Links with the Local Community

Dorit Braun

Why continuing consultation?

Maternity services users, uniquely amongst most users of services, give everyone an opportunity for insight, understanding and feedback on a whole range of other services since all the literature demonstrates that women are the chief health carers of their families. By consulting with users of maternity services on a continuing basis, you have, therefore, a way into views about child health services, about primary healthcare services generally for families and even about services for older people, as child bearing women might also be caring for parents or other relatives.

Where will we find people?

If we want to develop continuing consultation with users and potential users of maternity services, it is important that we develop good working relationships with them; and so where we look for people and how we engage them in the first instance is of critical importance.

There are some obvious places to find users of maternity services, for example:

- Antenatal clinics
- GPs
- Hospitals
- Well baby clinics
- Toddler groups

If you want to find people who are willing to talk to you about more than the health service aspects of their care, look for places where people are doing things other than being looked after because they are pregnant, or just about to give birth, or have just given birth. Look for instance in play groups, schools, nurseries and perhaps even churches, supermarkets, chemists, libraries and other public places.

Who are we trying to contact?

It is important to recognise that some groups do worse out of current systems of health care than others. Purchasers, need to look at people who appear not to be benefiting from current services and try to find out why. There is nothing wrong in having a bias when looking for people to consult, towards people who traditionally do not do well from services, or find it difficult to access them. Black and ethnic minority women from the various communities where you work may well be a priority for consultation and for continuing consultation. Similarly, families living on council housing estates, families with low incomes, or where someone is unemployed may be of particular interest to you. These people are traditionally the ones who are hardest to reach. However there are ways they can be reached through working with organisations who are already in touch with such communities. Black run organisations which have contact with members of their community, may assist you in reaching those groups.

Similarly, nursery schools, health visitors, housing advice workers, even welfare rights workers are likely to have some contact with many of the kinds of people you might want to consult. However, if you are going to try to achieve meaningful consultation with hard to reach groups, you need to do it with help from people who are working closely with such groups.

The Northampton experience

Northamptonshire has been developing a purchasing strategy for services for people with physical disabilities, between the FHSA, social services, the voluntary sector and the health authority. This has involved an extensive consultation exercise with users of services and with black and ethnic minority communities, commissioned from an appropriate organisation. A consumer group which is part of the Council for the Disabled in Northamptonshire, has undertaken the consultation with users across the county and a black community leader has undertaken work using linkworkers and other community organisations to find black disabled people and involve them in the consultation exercise. It is important to recognise that this work costs money. Community organisations and voluntary groups who are struggling for resources can not be expected to undertake proper consultation exercises for free. However, it has not been overly expensive; something in the region of £26,000 has been spent on both pieces of consultation. The pay-off has been that there are something like 400 or 500 people across the county who have been actively involved in developing the strategy and who will continue to be there for us to go back to them, when we need to monitor how effectively it is being implemented.

Some pitfalls to avoid

Firstly, the relationships which we develop with the people we are consulting are absolutely critical. Therefore, we should not get hung up about doing scientific, 'hard' research. We should instead concentrate on how to develop good, productive relationships based on mutual understanding and trust. This seems to me to necessitate a qualitative approach to research. This does not mean that we should not count the number of people with whom we have been in contact, or even count and categorise some of their responses to issues which they have raised so that we get a sense of quantity. We should not abandon counting and quantitative work but we should recognise that the focus of continuing consultation is bound to be qualitative because of the nature of the involvement that we are seeking.

The second pitfall, which is infinitely more likely to trap us than using the wrong kind of research method, is that we find ourselves completely unable to act on the feedback we receive from consultation. There is nothing worse than undertaking research with consumers of our services and then failing to do anything about the things they tell us. If we invest carefully in developing good relationships with people, their networks and grass roots links will pay dividends in terms of enabling us to keep going back and developing good, constructive working relationships. Similarly if we fail to respond to the things they are saying to us it will take us years to recover our credibility. For this reason it is absolutely crucial that before you go and consult anyone about anything you need to be clear about the mechanismsyou will use for dealing with the feedback that you are going to get. The time involved in negotiating who is responsible for consultation and what is going to happen to the feedback should not be underestimated.

Conclusion

It is important to recognise that many of the changes that consumers ask for do not cost huge amounts of money but do require enormous shifts in attitudes, values and the ways that services are provided by professionals. If we find it difficult to implement these changes or fund them, at the very least we owe it to consumers to explain what our difficulties are. They may well be in a position to help in terms of training sessions, talking directly to staff and supporting the shift in attitudes. The value of continuing consultation is not only that relationships become more equal but that both users and health professionals benefit from the relationship.

Dorit Braun
Locality Purchasing Local Community Co-ordinator
Northants Health Authority

The Case for Maternity Services Liaison Committees

Helen Lewison

Maternity Services Liaison Committees (MSLC) are unique in the NHS. Devised by the Maternity Services Advisory Committee[1] in the early 1980s, they provide a forum for representatives from all groups with an interest in maternity care, including users, to meet regularly and advise district health authorities on all aspects of local maternity services[2,3]. As advisory groups, they are dependent on the commitment of both the purchasing authority and providers to act on decisions made by the committee. Constituted properly and chaired efficiently, they can act as a clearing-house for all matters to do with maternity services. Uniquely, they offer users the opportunity to influence the planning and monitoring of services at district health authority level.

One of the objectives of *Changing Childbirth*[4] is that: 'users of maternity services should be actively involved in planning and reviewing services. The lay representation must reflect the ethnic, cultural and social mix of the local population. A MSLC should be established within every district health authority.' It also states that, 'The MSLC, chaired by a lay person, should report primarily to the purchasers but will also need to refer to providers on local issues. Purchasers need to ensure that a MSLC is established within each purchasing authority and should also agree the committee's constitution and remit.'

The chapter in *Changing Childbirth* entitled 'Action for Change' contains no specific role for the MSLC. However, it is difficult to see what other body has sufficient representation from all stakeholders in maternity services to plan, own, oversee the implementation of and monitor the changes required in order to meet the aims, objectives and indicators of success set out in *Changing Childbirth*.

MSLCs in the past have had a very bad press from many health professionals, managers and users[5]. In particular, MSLCs were often regarded, and indeed still are by some, as being ineffective. It is suggested that the principal reasons for this are that many of them were badly constituted, poorly managed and provider based and dominated. Often their function was to indicate what was in fact only a token consultation of users. It is significant that in the past the tendency of some district health authorities was to side-step local MSLCs (there might often be one in each provider unit), by setting up *ad hoc* groups to carry out the 'real work' of radical reviews and strategic planning of maternity services.

It is suggested that this energy might be better deployed by purchasing authorities setting up properly constituted MSLCs with representation from all relevant stakeholders, so that a standing advisory group is available to advise, plan and monitor all aspects of maternity services on a permanent basis. Sub-groups, both standing and *ad hoc*, including co-opted members when necessary, can be set up to carry out more detailed work and special projects under the auspices of and accountable to the MSLC. These could include sub-groups located at provider level with user representation to work on issues pertinent solely to providers.

The main strength of the MSLC is its multi-disciplinary nature, allowing all stakeholders to own the process of change. Its main weakness is its dependence on the commitment and goodwill both of its participants to make it work and the purchasing authority and providers to act on the results of the MSLC's deliberations.

One thorny problem is that of user representation: how possible is it for the sort of people able to participate effectively in a large, formal committee composed principally of health professionals and managers, to represent all users, particularly those whose voice is rarely heard in any forum? There is no doubt that the detailed work of influencing the contracting and other NHS processes has to take place in a formal committee, with all that entails. Ideally, all relevant groups of local users, including women from black and ethnic minority groups and those with disabilities or with special needs, would be represented in this way and perhaps they eventually will be. But where women from these groups are unable or unwilling to take part in these formal processes for the time being, other ways have to be found of making sure that their views are heard. Already many district health authorities have set up maternity services user groups, composed of women who have recently had babies, to pass on their views to user representatives. In turn, the user representatives have to be accountable to the groups and show that they have taken appropriate issues to the MSLC. Different mechanisms have been found for different communities with diverse populations and, doubtless, more could be, and are, being created all the time.

The Greater London Association of Community Health Councils (GLACHC) has recently obtained a grant from the Department of Health *Changing Childbirth* implementation monies to develop and evaluate a scheme for training current and potential user representatives on MSLCs. As well as regular peer support groups and training days, reference groups composed of women from a wide range of backgrounds will meet to inform the user representatives and, it is hoped, inspire some of these women with the confidence to themselves take on the role of representing childbearing women in their communities on their MSLC.

Thus there is a place for consultation with users at several different levels in order to ensure that the MSLC truly represents their views and is accountable to them. Potentially, the MSLC could be used as a model in other fields of health care for involving many different groups of users.

Helen Lewison
NCT member

References

1. Department of Health (1982, 1984, 1985). *Maternity Care in Action* - Parts 1, 2 and 3 Crown Copyright.
2. Garcia, J. (1987). 'The role and structure of the MSLC' *Health Trends*, Vol 19 pp 17-19.
3. Royal College of Midwives (1992). *Survey of Maternity Services Liaison Committees* (unpublished).
4. Department of Health (1993). *Changing Childbirth*, London: HMSO.
5. Newburn, M. (1992). 'Participation in policy-making: the maternity service users' in Ed Chamberlain, G., Zander, L. *Pregnancy Care in the 1990s Proceedings of a symposium held at the Royal Society of Medicine Parthenon.*

Editors Note:Helen Lewison has written an extensive briefing paper on MSLCs entitled 'MSLCs A Forum for Change'available from GLACHC, 356 Holloway Road ,London N7 6PA.

Strengthening the User Voice on MSLCs

Gillian Fletcher

Introduction

Changing Childbirth recommends that the first principle of the maternity services should be that 'The woman must be the focus of maternity care. She should be able to feel that she is in control of what is happening to her and able to make decisions about her care, based on her needs, having discussed matters fully with the professionals involved.'

The experience of one MSLC

Members of the East Surrey Maternity Services Liaison Committee have, like many other people involved in the maternity services in England, been thinking about ways in which we can begin to implement the recommendations of *Changing Childbirth* in our area. Working through the recommendations we were pleased to find that many of them are already happening in our maternity unit. We are conscious of the need to avoid any complacency and, looking at ways of implementing the remaining recommendations, we decided we needed to increase consumer representation on the MSLC. This committee consists of many health professionals and a few lay representatives and is already a large committee. We decided that it would be much more fruitful to have a separate sub-group of consumers which would meet every six weeks, as does the MSLC, so that information could be readily fed from one group to the other. The main benefit of this arrangement is that we can have more consumer representatives than we could accommodate on the main committee, and they might feel more relaxed within their own peer group than they might feel on a committee dominated by health professionals.

As well as electing a chair of the MSLC and revising the terms of reference, we decided to go ahead in early 1994 and set up the consumer sub group. Posters and flyers were distributed around the hospital and clinics and midwives were encouraged to draw people's attention to these.

Our poster uses a format similar to the one for our Antenatal Day Care Drop-In Unit which received a mention in Part II of *Changing Childbirth* as an example of clear and simple communication. We advertised details of two open meetings in the local press and on local radio. We were a little disappointed but undaunted by the poor attendance at the open meetings and decided to go ahead with the first meeting of the group in April 1994 at which we had six people, two couples and two women without their partners, plus the Director of Midwifery, me as the lay Chair of the MSLC and one small baby. Most of this first meeting was taken up with getting to know a little about one another which was important in order to create a relaxed and open climate where people would not be afraid to speak openly.

We needed to find out what their expectations for the group were, outline the way we had envisaged the group might work and set some groundrules and agenda items for future meetings. We did this by asking them to list items under the four G's.

- Gives
- Gets
- Ghastlies
- Groundrules

I find this is a useful exercise to do with any new group to help them focus on how they might function and to help us all recognise and value the contributions they have to make. It also helps highlight any fears or anxieties people may have about belonging to a new group if they are not entirely clear, initially, about its function.

What users give to a group
- Recent personal experience
- Experience of others through their contacts at clinics, coffee mornings, mother and baby groups etc.
- Wide and differing viewpoints,
- Suggestions for improvements
- Open minds

What users get from a group
- Learning from others
- A feeling of making a contribution
- Knowledge that they may have helped to avoid mistakes being made in the future
- A sense of achievement in contributing to improvements in the services locally.

What users dread in groups
- Unknown commitment
- Inhibitions at meetings,
- Fear that it could turn into one big 'whinge session' (this was a fear we shared)
- Meetings would be too long winded and possibly focusing on trivialities,

Ground rules for working in groups

- Time keeping - everyone's responsibility
- Agenda setting in advance to make maximum use of the time available at meetings
- Joint responsibility for running of the group
- Freedom to raise issues and concerns
- Let's not get too heavy in our discussions
- Valuing everyone's contributions
- Listening to each other

We felt this to be a very positive start to our group's life and after some discussion about items for the next agenda they left with the task of reviewing all the information they had received during pregnancy. What, when it was received from whom and where it had been obtained and to come back with recommendations for improvement.

They were very committed and at the next meeting we filled a flip chart page with their ideas for improvements.

We have since had three more meetings and are currently actively recruiting more members, trying to get people with a broad range of experiences of using the services.

Composition of the group

We have members in early pregnancy, those with very small babies and older babies up to a year old, someone whose baby was born very prematurely transferred to a regional intensive care baby unit and then back to our own special care baby unit, someone who has infertility treatment, someone who had twins, one of whom was sadly stillborn.

A couple who are both profoundly deaf have offered to give us written feedback about how the services met their specific needs with any suggestions for improvements.

We envisage that members will stay on the group until their baby is about nine months to a year old, when they will be replaced by others who are currently using the maternity services. Those who join in early pregnancy may stay on the group for up to 18 months.

We are conscious of the need to recruit consumers from all the areas of our health district as well as from many different socio-economic and ethic groups. We are also aware of the need to look at other ways of getting feedback from people who may not feel this group is for them - such as the couple who are deaf, or teenagers who are pregnant.

Feedback

The feedback we have had from the group members has been that generally people are happy with the services they have received/are receiving but they have certainly made a number of really useful suggestions which are now being implemented. Three midwives have been given the task of taking forward the suggestions which are now being implemented. Three midwives have been given the task of taking forward the suggestions and reporting back on progress to the group at each meeting. Other suggestions and comments are taken back to the MSLC for discussion or implementation. Any of the group members are very welcome to attend the MSLC meetings at any time and the two lay members of the MSLC and the Director of Midwifery attend the consumer group meetings. Any new leaflets which are being planned will be piloted through the consumer group first, in order to get the level and amount of information right according to those who use that information rather than those who provide the service deciding, in isolation, what information they think women need.

Conclusions

Many people find change difficult. It is always likely to be slower that you had anticipated and of course financial constraints have always to be taken into consideration but I am finding it very exciting to be involved in this process of change and improvement. As an NCT teacher and tutor of 23 years I have at times felt exceedingly frustrated at how slowly things can be changed for the better. Over the years I have received feedback from women after the birth of their baby about situations which they found extremely demoralising and distressing and I realised that while the medical care and expertise has often been excellent, it was the patronising attitude and lack of dignity and respect for feelings and wishes that led to the experience being so negative for the woman. The frustration came from not being able to change that. With the publication of *Changing Childbirth* and the new focus so clearly needing to be on the feelings and wishes of the woman and her partner. At last attitudes are beginning to change.

Gillian Fletcher,
NCT member

Editors Note: This paper is reproduced with the permission of the Newsletter for the Association of Community Based Maternity Care.

Listening with Mother - Some Concluding Remarks

Karlene Davis

The papers in this collection are all about how purchasers and providers can more effectively consult users of the maternity services. The aim has been to provide the beginnings of a tool-kit to use in units and authorities, to look again at how you are doing 'it', and whether you can do 'it' better.

To conclude the collection, it may be helpful to return to first principles - *why should you even bother consulting users of the maternity (or indeed any) services?*

Because it is important if consultation is going to be meaningful and worthwhile, that those doing it should not only understand 'how', but also believe in what they are doing.

Some of the philosophical and pragmatic reasons that emerge in the course of this collection include:

- Firstly, I think we can agree that in all democratic societies there is an understanding that those who contribute to or use a service should have some control over it. Users of the maternity services are paying for the service - they are paying our salaries - it is therefore only right that we are accountable to them.

- Secondly, in the NHS environment, purchasers and providers have to face the fact that users will when they are given the opportunity exercise choice. Effectively competing in the health service market means not only knowing what the competition is offering, but also what the customer wants.

- Thirdly, *Changing Childbirth* is Government policy: it includes targets which are to be met within five years and the NHS Executive has made it clear that individual managers' performance assessment will include the speed and effectiveness of implementation.

- Next, participation is one way of maximising the efficiency of health services by increasing compliance and utilisation. For example, greater cultural sensitivity reflecting real needs is likely to pay dividends in promoting the adoption of healthier lifestyles.

and finally,

- Participation is a prerequisite to a successful health care market. Health service users or consumers must have sufficient information to make rational decisions in the health market.

As this collection has shown, the whole issue of the role that users play within policy development and their place in the delivery of care has grown enormously in the last ten years. Local and national groups have become increasingly sophisticated and effective in articulating users demands and representing their interests. Some of these groups are very familiar, others perhaps less so:

- Community Health Councils
- Patients' Association
- College of Health
- Action for Victims of Medical Accidents
- Health Rights
- National Association for Patient Participation

Within the maternity services, the explosion of voluntary and self-help groups must lead us to examine whether we have failed to provide appropriate, sensitive and relevant services. There are groups such as:

- Association for Improvements in Maternity Services
- Pre-Eclamptic Toxaemia Society
- Stillbirth and Neonatal Death Society
- Toxoplasmosis Trust
- Twins and Multiple Births Association.

These groups all share a belief that health services should be run for the benefit of those who use them rather than those who work in them.

For some, this might be quite a challenging concept, and perhaps it is time to ask whether we are really committed to involving users, or are we merely paying lip service?

One way to address this through the contractual process is actually to define what we mean by

- Patients' rights
- Patients' satisfaction
- Patient participation

The Patients Charter and the Maternity Charter set out a framework of rights that purchasers and providers can work within, but can these be extended?

Patient satisfaction is now recognised as an important outcome measure within the audit process, but how well is it being measured?

The title of this collection: 'Listen with Mother' implies that both rights and satisfaction can only be properly addressed through participation - actually involving users. There is a place for users at every stage of the contractual process and it is to the advantage of purchasers and providers to involve users in:

- Assessing local health needs
- Appraising service options
- Choosing patterns of delivery
- Placing contracts
- Monitoring contracts
- Renewing contracts

Conclusions

One of the key messages which has emerged is the importance of promoting both formal and informal consultation, through existing networks and by establishing new ones. The papers on consulting hard to reach groups and continuing consultation are about achieving genuine representation. There is already a body of literature to assist in this process, from the Commission for Racial Equality's recent Code of Practice for the Maternity Services to the RCM's guidelines on Maternity Services Liaison Committees. There is, of course, a great deal more and many of the consumer groups who are represented here today have produced their own guidelines - so none of us needs to reinvent the wheel.

The second major issue which deserves highlighting from the papers on research methodologies is that we are still basing services on our notions of 'what women want'. But 'what women want' is as diverse as women themselves - it cannot be captured in glib phrases, we have got to make the effort to undertake relevant research. This means finding out what users really think, not what midwives say women want, and not what obstetricians, GPs, or managers say women want. We must allow women - all women to speak for themselves.

Karlene Davis
Deputy General Secretary
Royal College of Midwives

Appendix

'I Wish I'd Known Before I Started...'

At the final Listen with Mother conference, we asked workshop leaders to offer a few warnings and practical tips to researchers starting out. The following points are drawn from their suggestions for quantitative or qualitative research....

Know your patch - Find out who's in your area - how they contact the maternity services - whether local organizations could help you approach them.

Think creatively - The maternity services may not be the most appropriate route to the women you want to reach - where else might you recruit them?

Take your time to plan - Some groups may be harder to reach than you thought - talk to others who have undertaken similar work or used similar techniques. Focus groups may not be the cheap option they appear, setting up and transcribing can be time-consuming. Review the literature.

Be flexible - Be prepared to meet women on their territory, make it easy for them to say what they really feel - offer practical support - a crèche may make all the difference to a group's functioning.

Have back up - Carry spare batteries, tapes etc., have someone take detailed notes whenever possible.

Get expert - Questionnaire design is hard - for example, too many open-ended questions may not be helpful

Get statistical advice - Consider what statistics you are likely to want before you design the research. Sample size, for example, will affect the level of confidence you can have in your conclusions.

Run a pilot - Test your questionnaire/interview schedule and take advice from people who know your target group, in and outside the maternity services. Frame preference questions in ways which allow people to think freely, without feeling constrained by experience or expectation: try 'If you could choose....'

'Clean the data' - Checking data for internal inconsistencies, completeness, legibility etc. before you begin analysis is time well spent.

Give feedback - Participants like to know what others have said, what conclusions you have come to and what you plan to do with the information they have provided.

... and specifically on influencing consultation through a maternity services liaison committee

Contact other MSLC's - Find out what they are doing and how successful they have been

Learn group skills - Basic group skills techniques are invaluable for meetings.

Understand the NHS - Find out how the NHS and the purchaser/provider split works locally and the implications for the functioning of the MSLC.

Keep calm - Don't get frustrated when progress is slow, build on small successes - changing attitudes and behaviour takes time.

Listen With Mother

Consulting Users of
Maternity Services

Edited by Rosemary Dodds, NCT,
Meg Goodman, MA and
Suzanne Tyler, RCM

Books for Midwives Press
Books for Midwives Press ... at collaboration
between the Royal Colle...   Midwives and
Haigh and Hochland ...   ...ations Ltd

Published by Books for Midwives Press, 174a Ashley Road, Hale, Cheshire, WA15 9SF, England

© 1996, Maternity Alliance

First edition

ISBN 1 898507 48 1

British Library Cataloguing in Publication Data
A catalogue record for this book is available from the British Library

Printed in Great Britain by The Cromwell Press Ltd